Experts' Perspectives on Medical Advances

This book series presents Chinese experts' perspectives on recent developments in clinical medicine. Written by leading Chinese experts in related fields, a wide variety of emerging and hot topics in internal medicine, surgery, oncology, neurosurgery, and ophthalmonology, etc., is covered by the series. Each title in this series covers a disease or a group of diseases, focusing on the basic knowledge, development and the latest research progress of clinical practice. This series is a practical and useful resource for researchers and practitioners in related subjects, as well as for general interest readers.

Lisheng Yu
Editor

Progress in Postauricular Administration

Springer

科学技术文献出版社
SCIENTIFIC AND TECHNICAL DOCUMENTATION PRESS

Editor
Lisheng Yu
Department of Otorhinolaryngology
Head and Neck Surgery, People's Hospital
Peking University
Beijing, China

ISSN 2948-1023 ISSN 2948-1031 (electronic)
Experts' Perspectives on Medical Advances
ISBN 978-981-95-5101-9 ISBN 978-981-95-5102-6 (eBook)
https://doi.org/10.1007/978-981-95-5102-6

Jointly published with Scientific and Technical Documentation Press
The print edition is not for sale in China (Mainland). Customers from China (Mainland) please order the print book from: Scientific and Technical Documentation Press.

Translation from the Chinese language edition: "耳科学余力生2021观点" by Lisheng Yu, © Scientific and Technical Documentation Press. Published by Scientific and Technical Documentation Press. 2021. All Rights Reserved.
The original submitted manuscript has been translated into English. The translation was done using artificial intelligence. A subsequent revision was performed by the author(s) to further refine the work and to ensure that the translation is appropriate concerning content and scientific correctness. It may, however, read stylistically different from a conventional translation.
Translation from the Chinese language edition: "耳科学余力生2021观点" by Lisheng Yu, © Scientific and Technical Documentation Press. Published by Scientific and Technical Documentation Press. 2021. All Rights Reserved.

This Springer imprint is published by the registered company Springer Nature Singapore Pte Ltd.
The registered company address is: 152 Beach Road, #21-01/04 Gateway East, Singapore 189721, Singapore

Contents

1 Otitis Media and the Middle Ear Ventilation System

Muhan Shi, Yujie Ke, Jilei Zhang, and Lisheng Yu

Otitis media is the most common inflammatory disease in otology. It is the most common cause for medical visits among children in the United States. Approximately 30 million pediatric visits occur annually in the United States, with over five million due to acute otitis media. Almost all children have had at least one episode of otitis media before the age of three, with more than half having experienced it three times or more. Helms suggests that most cases of chronic suppurative otitis media and acquired cholesteatoma in adults begin in childhood. Surgery for otitis media is the most common reason for general anesthesia in children, with annual treatment costs in the United States exceeding five million US dollars. Otitis media is the most common cause of acquired hearing loss in children. It is more prevalent in winter and less common in summer [1]. Some studies indicate that the incidence rate is higher in males than in females. There is no significant difference in the incidence of otitis media between White and Black children in the United States [2]. However, the incidence is higher among Native Americans and Alaska Natives (Eskimos). The incidence of chronic suppurative otitis media in industrialized countries (such as the United States and the UK) is less than 1%. This indicates that social hygiene conditions have a significant impact on chronic otitis media. About one-third are bilateral cases.

The 2004 guidelines for the diagnosis and treatment of otitis media in China classified chronic suppurative otitis media into three types: simple type (lesions limited to the mucosa), osteitis type (involving the bone), and cholesteatoma type. Since some middle ear cholesteatomas are not significantly related to inflammation, the 2012 guidelines for the diagnosis and treatment of otitis media in China listed middle ear cholesteatoma separately. Internationally, there is no such term as "osteitis-type otitis media," but rather it is referred to as "chronic mastoiditis."

It has long been believed that Eustachian tube dysfunction is the main cause of nonsuppurative otitis media (secretory otitis media), while infection is the main cause of suppurative otitis media. Bacterial cultures of effusion specimens from secretory otitis media (*Haemophilus influenzae*, *Streptococcus pneumoniae*, and *Moraxella catarrhalis*) have a positive rate of only 30–40%, but a large amount of inflammatory mediators are found in chronic effusions. Extensive pathological studies of otitis media temporal bones show that in early otitis media (including acute otitis media) and chronic otitis media, purulent effusions account for 75% and 56.3%, respectively, but most do not have obvious symptoms of otitis media, and the tympanic membrane is intact. Therefore, it is difficult to distinguish secretory otitis media from purulent otitis media with no

M. Shi · Y. Ke · J. Zhang · L. Yu (✉)
Department of Otorhinolaryngology, Head and Neck Surgery, People's Hospital, Peking University, Beijing, China

L. Yu (ed.), *Progress in Postauricular Administration*, Experts' Perspectives on Medical Advances, https://doi.org/10.1007/978-981-95-5102-6_1

obvious symptoms based solely on clinical symptoms.

Post (1995) used polymerase chain reaction (PCR) technology to study samples from 97 cases of secretory otitis media and found that only 28 cases (28.9%) were positive for *Haemophilus influenzae*, *Streptococcus pneumoniae*, and *Moraxella catarrhalis* by all three methods of bacterial culture and PCR [3]. However, in 75 cases (77.3%), one or more types of bacteria were positive by PCR, while all three bacterial cultures were negative. Rayner et al. (1998) used reverse transcriptase PCR to detect *Haemophilus influenzae* and found that bacteria in the middle ear effusion actively synthesized mRNA, indicating that the bacteria were viable, functional, and metabolically active [4]. Dingman et al. (1998) found that endotoxins in chronic middle ear effusions were highly correlated with *Haemophilus influenzae* and *Moraxella catarrhalis*, which could be detected by PCR but showed no bacterial growth in culture [5]. In 50 children with secretory otitis media, after tympanostomy tube placement, examinations using bacterial culture, PCR, in situ hybridization, immunofluorescence staining, and confocal laser scanning microscopy (CLSM) combined with bacterial live-dead staining methods revealed biofilms in 46 cases. All 27 effusions tested positive for at least 1 pathogen that can cause otitis media by PCR (*Haemophilus influenzae*, *Streptococcus pneumoniae*, *Moraxella catarrhalis*), but only 6 of the 27 cases (22%) had positive bacterial cultures for any of the bacteria. This indicates that determining the bacterial environment in the middle ear based on bacterial culture results has significant limitations. It also suggests that biofilms can be seen in the remission period of recurrent otitis media in children, indicating that bacteria are not eliminated during the intermission of acute episodes [6]. The disease process is not driven by inflammatory mediators but is the result of persistent bacteria. The presence of biofilms has been confirmed in middle ear effusions and repeated episodes of otitis media in middle ear mucosal sections using confocal laser scanning microscopy, which were not found in the control group of normal middle ear cavities. In such cases, the positive rate of bacterial culture is very low. Due to the presence of biofilms, there is high antibiotic resistance, so monotherapy with antibiotics is often not effective.

Gibson (1994), Tasker (2002), and Velepic (2000) believe that otitis media is related to gastroesophageal diseases [7–9]. Tasker (2002) used enzyme-linked immunosorbent assay and enzyme activity tests to measure the concentration of pepsin in children's middle ear effusions, finding 83% positivity (45/54 cases). In another study by Tasker (2002), the levels of pepsin and pepsinogen in the middle ear effusions of 65 children were measured, and 59 cases had levels more than 1000 times higher than serum, which is considered to be caused by gastric acid reflux [10]. Poelmans et al. (2002) found a correlation between adult effusive otitis media or Eustachian tube dysfunction and gastric acid reflux, and treatment with antireflux drugs was effective, but it was not a randomized clinical trial [11].

Bluestone believes that middle ear effusion is the fluid produced by otitis media, which can be serous, mucoid, or purulent [12]. Persistent middle ear effusion is the persistent fluid in the middle ear after an acute episode of otitis media. Chronic otitis media and chronic suppurative otitis media are synonymous. According to the guidelines for the diagnosis and treatment of otitis media established in China in 2012, otitis media is divided into secretory and purulent otitis media. As can be seen from the above research results, it is actually difficult to define secretory (nonsuppurative) otitis media and purulent otitis media in clinical practice. A negative bacterial culture does not mean the absence of pathogens but is due to the backwardness of previous detection methods. Transudate, exudate, secretion, glue ear, and suppuration are just different pathological processes in otitis media, and any single link cannot reflect the whole picture of the disease. The term used abroad is "otitis media with effusion" instead of "secretory otitis media." Therefore, the accurate translation is recommended to be "effusion otitis media." Continuing to use the concept of "secretory otitis media" is not only inaccurate but also misleading.

Therefore, the basic principle of otitis media treatment, in addition to the use of antibiotics (which is often ineffective due to the presence of biofilms), is to ensure smooth drainage. The basic surgical principle for chronic suppurative otitis media is to improve ventilation and drainage and to preserve or reconstruct function (hearing function, treatment of the posterior wall of the external auditory canal, etc.). The focus is on drainage! Therefore, it is essential to understand the ventilation and drainage system of the middle ear. The first step is to understand the structure and function of the Eustachian tube.

1.1 The History and Structure of the Eustachian Tube

The Italian Bartolomeus Eustachius first described the auditory tube (Eustachian tube) in his 1562 doctoral thesis, *Epistola de auditus organis*: There is an auditory passage, known as the concha, in the tympanic cavity of the petrous part of the temporal bone, which perforates toward the nasal cavity. Eustachius not only described the anatomical structure but also introduced its physiological and therapeutic importance. His discovery was not taken seriously until the nineteenth century. Antonio Maria Valsalva (1666–1723) provided a classic description of the Eustachian tube in his work *Treatise on the Human Ear*, detailing the cartilage, membrane, and bony parts of the tube. He discovered the tensor veli palatini muscle and called it the tube dilator muscle. He believed the Eustachian tube had an acoustic function, supported the idea of draining purulent material from the middle ear, invented the Valsalva maneuver to treat middle ear effusion and negative pressure, and also used it as an inflation test for tube patency. The British physician Joseph Toynbee (1815–1866) invented the Toynbee test. Adam Politzer (1835–1920), the most famous otologist of the nineteenth century and recognized as the father of modern otology, invented the Eustachian tube insufflation method, which is still in use today. His theory on the role of the Eustachian tube in the pathogenesis of middle ear effusion, the hydrops ex vacuo of serous fluid, is still considered a correct explanation: "Undoubtedly, sometimes the excessive swelling and impermeability of the mucous membrane of the Eustachian tube, due to the continuous thinning of the air in the tympanic cavity, lead to the transudation of serous fluid."

The Eustachian tube is the passage connecting the middle ear to the nasopharynx. In adults, the Eustachian tube is about 31–38 mm long, with the outer one-third being bony and the inner two-thirds cartilaginous. The connecting part between the two is called the isthmus, which is the narrowest part of the tube. The area of the isthmus is relatively stable among different individuals, while the areas of the pharyngeal and tympanic orifices vary. The pharyngeal orifice is 7.37 mm^2 ± 5.65 mm^2, the isthmus 0.65 mm^2 ± 20.19 mm^2, and the tympanic orifice 18.63 mm^2 ± 5.48 mm^2. The diameter of the isthmus decreases, and in infancy, the length of the Eustachian tube is only half that of an adult, averaging 18 mm, and it reaches the adult size by the age of seven, mainly due to the development of the bony part. The course of the Eustachian tube is not a straight line but a slightly curved reverse "S" shape.

The main physiological functions of the Eustachian tube are the following:

(1) Ventilation function: It opens about 1.4 times per minute, lasting 0.4–0.5 s.
(2) Drainage and removal of secretions produced in the middle ear to the nasopharynx.
(3) Protective function: Preventing gastroesophageal reflux from entering the middle ear, preventing sound from entering the tympanic cavity when speaking.

The main role of the Eustachian tube in the middle ear ventilation system is to open for ventilation and to clear.

The middle ear ventilation system consists of the Eustachian tube (active muscle opening mechanism, mucociliary mechanism at the tympanic orifice of the tube), the tympanic membrane pressure receptors, the cochlear promontory chemical receptors, the second valve (around the malleus), the anterior and posterior isthmuses of the epitympanic and mesotympanic spaces, the middle ear pressure regulation system, etc.

1.2 The Opening Function of the Eustachian Tube

In the first half of the twentieth century, Arnold Rice Rich, a professor at Johns Hopkins Medical School, conducted research on the physiology of the muscles related to the Eustachian tube (tensor veli palatini, tensor tympani, levator veli palatini, and pharyngeal constrictor muscles) and surrounding structures and concluded that the tensor veli palatini is the most significant factor in the active dilation of the Eustachian tube. In the mid-twentieth century, H. B. Perlman from the University of Chicago discovered that denervation of the tensor veli palatini can lead to abnormal patency of the Eustachian tube. Building on the research of his predecessors, Bluestone was the first to propose the view that "the Eustachian tube is not a simple passage but an independent organ," composed of the lumen mucosa, cartilage, surrounding soft tissue, tube-adjacent muscles (tensor veli palatini, levator veli palatini, tensor tympani, pharyngeal constrictor muscles), and bony support. The tensor veli palatini, tensor tympani, levator veli palatini, and pharyngeal constrictor muscles, each muscle has a time related to the function of the Eustachian tube. The tube is passively closed at rest. It opens during swallowing, yawning, and sneezing. The tensor veli palatini is attached only to the cartilaginous part of the Eustachian tube, and most anatomical and physiological evidence supports that the active dilation of the Eustachian tube is due to the action of the tensor veli palatini or with the assistance of the levator veli palatini. The closure of the tube mainly depends on the pressure of the surrounding deforming tissue of the tube wall, and the tube wall is passively closed under the combined action of the rebound of the elastic fibers inside the cartilage. Under normal circumstances, the bony part of the Eustachian tube is always open in a healthy state, and the cartilaginous part is closed at rest, only opening passively during swallowing and yawning due to the contraction of the tensor veli palatini, with an opening frequency of 1000 times a day. This intermittent opening is very significant for maintaining normal middle ear function. It is estimated that the normal opening time of the Eustachian tube is about 400 milliseconds, with about one swallow per minute when awake and one swallow every 5 min during sleep. The normal Eustachian tube is closed at rest, and when swallowing, the tensor veli palatini contracts; the proximal part of the cartilaginous part opens first, followed by the expansion of the distal part of the tube; after active dilation, the tube passively shrinks back to the resting position (closed); the sequence is reversed, starting from the distal end and then reaching the proximal end: this is very important for the clearing function of the Eustachian tube.

1.2.1 Eustachian Tube Dysfunction (Disorder)

In June 2014, medical experts and scientists in the field of Eustachian tube function research reached a consensus on the definition of Eustachian tube dysfunction, stating that it is caused by a disorder in the regulation of middle ear pressure and is divided into acute and chronic types. The course of the disease is less than 3 months for the acute type and more than 3 months for the chronic type. According to the form of the dysfunction, it can be divided into three subtypes: delayed opening-type Eustachian tube dysfunction, pressure-type Eustachian tube dysfunction, and abnormal opening of the Eustachian Tube. Since the focus of clinical research at home and abroad is mainly on the delayed opening type, it is further divided into three types: functional obstruction, dynamic obstruction, and anatomical obstruction.

Whether it is an opening type of Eustachian tube dysfunction or abnormal opening of the Eustachian tube, they are the final results of multiple causes. Finding the underlying causes is the key basis for treatment. Acute delayed opening-type Eustachian tube dysfunction is often caused by allergic diseases and upper respiratory tract infections that lead to the narrowing or even obstruction of the pharyngeal opening and tube of the Eustachian tube, resulting in poor ventilation of the Eustachian tube. The course of this type is relatively short, and the above symptoms will disappear as the causes of acute inflammation and allergic diseases are eliminated. The pathophysiological mechanism of chronic delayed opening-type Eustachian tube dysfunction is not yet fully clear.

1.2.2 Abnormal Opening of the Eustachian Tube

(See Section 3 of Objective Tinnitus: Objective Tinnitus of Respiratory Origin)

1.3 The Clearance Function of the Eustachian Tube (Mucous Excretion Mechanism)

The pharyngeal orifice of the Eustachian tube is innervated by branches of the otic ganglion, the sphenopalatine nerve, and the pharyngeal plexus. Sensory nerves for the rest of the Eustachian tube come from the tympanic plexus and the pharyngeal plexus. The glossopharyngeal nerve may play a primary role in the innervation of the Eustachian tube. The tensor veli palatini (and tensor tympani) are innervated by the trigeminal nerve (mandibular branch). The levator veli palatini does not primarily participate in the dilation of the Eustachian tube but has an auxiliary role. It may be more related to the pump clearance (drainage) function, helping to pump out the exudate from the middle ear.

The typical middle ear mucosal epithelium, especially near the tympanic orifice of the Eustachian tube, is composed of three layers of cells. The surface layer consists of mucus cells and ciliated cells intermingled, which is the basis of the function of the middle ear mucosal epithelium. Under normal conditions, mucus cells only appear around the tympanic orifice of the Eustachian tube. The cilia of ciliated cells swing rhythmically, and the mucus from mucus cells forms a mucus blanket on the surface of the mucosal cells, forming a mucus-ciliary clearance system in the middle ear cavity.

Leclerc (1987) found that the mucous membrane of the Eustachian tube has autonomous regulatory periodic fluctuations, similar to the nasal mucosa cycle [13]. Sando (1994) proposed a hypothesis through the study of temporal bone specimens: the upper part of the Eustachian tube lumen is related to the pressure regulation of the middle ear, and the lower part is responsible for clearance, both parts are related to the protective function of the middle ear [14]. Sade (1987) found that the clearance function was most active in the front half to two-thirds of the middle ear cavity by dripping reagents into the perforated eardrum of patients, and most studies show that the clearance function is related to the obstruction of the clearance of middle ear effusion, but it is not the main reason [15]. However, Shikowitz and others (1988) found that when there is a ciliary movement disorder in the upper respiratory tract mucosa, there is middle ear effusion.

The epitympanic area and the entrance of the tympanic antrum, the mastoid area, often do not have this mucus-ciliary clearance system to help clear the accumulated keratin and cannot be passively cleared like open skin, where shed keratin can be passively cleared. The middle ear cavity is mostly closed most of the time and only occasionally opens (such as during swallowing), so it is difficult to expel shed cells. Honjo found that when the volume of middle ear fluid is small, it is cleared by the mucociliary system; when the volume of fluid is large and the viscosity is low, it is cleared by muscle activity; high-viscosity fluid is cleared by both ciliary and muscle mechanisms [16]. And the clearance time is affected by the viscosity of the fluid in the mastoid rather than in the tympanic cavity, and the tympanic cavity is easier to clear than the mastoid.

Cholesteatomas are generally caused by functional obstruction of the Eustachian tube rather than mechanical (anatomical) obstruction. Recent studies generally believe that the possibility of pathological mechanical obstruction of the Eustachian tube causing otitis media is very small. Sade's measurement comparison of the cross-sectional area of the Eustachian tube lumen between otitis media temporal bones and normal temporal bones showed no significant difference, and all otitis media temporal bones had a patent Eustachian tube lumen, with no pathological mechanical obstruction [17]. These studies suggest that the Eustachian tube is not easily obstructed by inflammatory lesions in the pathological process of otitis media.

Zhang Quan'an found in the examination of 32 otitis media temporal bone specimens that the isthmus of the Eustachian tube was completely patent, with no pathological obstruction [18]. Inflammatory cell infiltration and vascular changes were very slight, close to normal. The thickness of the mucocartilaginous membrane was not significantly different from the normal group. The thickness of the mucoosseous membrane at the promontory was 6.51 times that of the normal group, and inflammatory cell infiltration and vascular changes were very significant. The mucocartilaginous membrane of the Eustachian tube and the mucoosseous membrane of the middle ear have completely different inflammatory responses to infection, and the clear boundary is exactly at the junction of the bone and cartilage of the Eustachian tube. Inflammatory lesions generally do not involve the mucocartilaginous membrane of the Eustachian tube, suggesting that the mucocartilaginous membrane of the cartilaginous part of the Eustachian tube has a strong barrier effect against inflammatory cell infiltration. Eustachian tube dysfunction is not the main cause of otitis media. On the contrary, during the course of otitis media, it is not obstructed by inflammatory lesions, and maintaining the patency of the ventilation and drainage channel is very beneficial for draining middle ear exudate and promoting the recovery of otitis media. The severe retraction of the eardrum may be related to the high negative pressure associated with middle ear effusion.

1.4 The Function and Surface-Active Substances of Eustachian Tube

The function of the Eustachian tube is related not only to the movement of surrounding muscles but also to the surface-active substances on the tube. The concept of surface-active substances on the Eustachian tube was first proposed by Fliesberg. Yang Weiyan and others observed the mucosal cells at the pharyngeal orifice of the Eustachian tube and confirmed the existence of surface-active substances there from a morphological perspective [19]. The top pleats of the Eustachian tube are mainly nonciliated cells that can secrete surface-active substances, which are mainly composed of phospholipids, polysaccharides, and proteins, similar to the components of pulmonary surfactant.

Surface-active substances on the Eustachian tube can help maintain its ventilation and clearance functions. Recent studies have shown that a deficiency of surface-active substances inside the Eustachian tube is one of the important causes of Eustachian tube dysfunction. Fornadley established a secretion otitis media model in hamsters and found that their Eustachian tube opening pressure increased [20]. After the injection of exogenous surface-active substances, their Eustachian tube opening pressure significantly decreased, suggesting that secretion otitis media is related to a decrease in surface-active substances. Nemechech conducted animal experiments with precise control of dosage and found that surface-active substances can effectively reduce the Eustachian tube opening pressure in experimental animals [21]. Treatment with surface-active substances can accelerate the improvement of secretory otitis media. Zhu Zhenghua proved that pulmonary surfactant administered through the nose can enter the Eustachian tube and exert its antiinflammatory effect on the mucous membrane ciliary system of the Eustachian tube in otitis media with effusion, protecting the ciliary structure [22].

1.4.1 The Impact of Pharyngeal Reflux on Surface-Active Substances of the Eustachian Tube

In animal experiments, White repeatedly washed the nasopharynx of rats with gastric juice, successfully inducing Eustachian tube dysfunction [23]. Different studies have mentioned that Eustachian tube dysfunction may be related to reflux, but the mechanism is unclear. Acute lung injury can cause a deficiency of surface-active substances, which is also one of the causes of acute respiratory distress syndrome, and an important cause of acute lung injury is the aspiration of gastric contents and/or respiratory system infection. Similarly, acidic gas-liquid reflux into the nasopharynx, passing through the Eustachian tube orifice by siphoning and other actions, may damage the surface-active substances in the nasopharynx and the Eustachian tube, significantly affecting the clearance and opening function of the Eustachian tube. Due to anatomical differences in the Eustachian tube between adults and children, reflux fluid in adults is relatively less likely to enter the Eustachian tube, thus reducing the proportion of secretory otitis media. However, the reduction of surface-active substances will affect the frequency and efficiency of the Eustachian tube's opening and closing, and patients often experience a feeling of ear stuffiness, which can also lead to the amplification of tinnitus signals, making them more likely to be transmitted to the auditory cortex and cause tinnitus.

From an anatomical perspective, there is a certain distance between the stomach and the nasopharynx. How does gastric juice reach the nasopharynx to affect the function of the Eustachian tube? The relaxation of the upper esophageal sphincter is the main cause of gas reflux. The esophagus and bronchial tree, which have the same embryonic origin, are both innervated by the vagus nerve. When gastric acid at the distal end of the esophagus stimulates the vagus nerve, it causes bronchoconstriction through reflexes, causing the patient to have repeated irritating coughs and throat-clearing actions, which is the main reason for promoting the jet of reflux liquid into the nasopharynx.

1.4.2 The Impact of Estrogen on Eustachian Tube Function

The impact of estrogen on Eustachian tube function is manifested in several aspects. First, the effects of estrogen and progesterone on nasal mucosa include local edema, gland hyperplasia, cellular infiltration, and increased vascular distribution, leading to symptomatic congestion of the nasal mucosa. The mucosa lining the Eustachian tube, like the nasal cavity and sinuses, is pseudostratified columnar ciliated respiratory epithelium. Sex hormones can cause congestion of the Eustachian tube mucosa, leading to functional disorders. Second, estrogen has a certain impact on surface-active substances in the Eustachian tube. During pregnancy, oral estrogen, or oral contraceptives, when the level of estrogen in the body increases, it increases the production of surface-active substances in the Eustachian tube, which is one of the reasons for the abnormal opening of the Eustachian tube. In postmenopausal women, the decline in estrogen levels may lead to a decrease in the secretion of surface-active substances in the Eustachian tube, resulting in poor opening.

1.5 The Role of the Tympanic Membrane

The presence of Schwann cells and axons in the tense part of the tympanic membrane is considered to be pressure receptors or stretch receptors. Research on normal subjects has confirmed this theory, indicating that they are mechanoreceptors for Eustachian tube function. After anesthesia of the tympanic membrane, a decrease in middle ear pressure may occur; hence the decline in Eustachian tube function is partly due to the reduced function of these pressure receptors. In cases of a complete perforation of the tympanic membrane, reconstruction may result in the loss of these pressure receptors, leading to Eustachian tube dysfunction. These pressure receptors are only found in the tense part of the tympanic membrane and play an important role in adjusting the function of the Eustachian tube. The tensor tympani muscle does not seem to be involved in the active opening of the Eustachian tube but can affect the opening function of the tensor veli palatini muscle through the pressure receptors of the tympanic membrane. An intact and undamaged tympanic membrane is crucial for Eustachian tube function; an incomplete tympanic membrane can impair the protective function of the Eustachian tube, leading to reflux of nasopharyngeal secretions. Conversely, Eustachian tube dysfunction can also adversely affect the tympanic membrane, such as in the case of tympanic membrane retraction. The physiological middle ear-mastoid gas cushion can help the Eustachian tube prevent reflux, aspiration, and insufflation of nasopharyngeal secretions. When a column of secretions enters the Eustachian tube toward the middle ear, the pressure in the mastoid of the middle ear becomes a higher positive pressure, acting as a cushion (gas pressure resistance). However, when there is a perforation of the tympanic membrane or a tympanic membrane tube in place, the cushion function is lost, and nasopharyngeal secretions can reflux into the middle ear.

1.6 The Chemical Receptors of the Tympanic Prominence

The neural innervation of the structures in the middle ear cavity comes from the branches of the tympanic plexus. Branches of the glossopharyngeal nerve: Jacobson's nerve (tympanic nerve). Eden and Ganon found that the tympanic plexus has neural connections with the ventral subnucleus of the ipsilateral solitary nucleus in the brainstem, speculating that this neural connection provides sensory input from chemical receptors in the middle ear, or pressure receptors, or both, which is related to the ventilation of the middle ear [24]. Shupak et al. reported that when the composition of gases in the middle ear changes, there is a difference in the ventilating function of the Eustachian tube, suggesting the presence of pressure receptors and/or chemical receptors in the middle ear [25]. It is speculated that the pressure receptors in the middle ear may be stimulated by signals from the stretch receptors of the tympanic membrane controlled by pressure changes in the external auditory canal. Thus, there may be a neuro-gas regulatory reflex arc in the tympanic prominence that can affect the ventilating function of the middle ear.

1.7 Ventilation of the Mastoid and Attic (The Second and Third Valves)

The middle ear ventilation system is a complex system, with the Eustachian tube being just one part, albeit an important component. Wullstein has long proposed that the area near the malleus is the site of the second valve of the middle ear. This area determines the ventilation and drainage of the tympanic antrum and most of the mastoid. The anterior and posterior isthmuses of the attic determine the drainage of the attic. Zhang Quan'an refers to the ventilation and drainage from the anterior middle ear cavity to the nasopharyngeal cavity as external ventilation drainage, and the ventilation and drainage from the mastoid cells through the antrum, tympanic isthmus, and umbilical-promontory isthmus (the narrow area between the umbo of the tympanic membrane and the promontory) to the anterior middle ear cavity as internal ventilation drainage [26]. As a result, among 290 temporal bone specimens of otitis media with inflammatory exudate (including serous, mucoid, and purulent exudates), the incidence of exudate accumulation in the anterior middle ear cavity was the lowest (47%), while the posterior middle ear cavity, attic, and tympanic antrum area were very high (88.6–96.2%). Granulation tissue in the anterior middle ear cavity was the least common (11.3%), while the formation rate of granulation tissue in the latter three areas was very high (86.4–90.7%). Takahashi found that the opening pressure of the Eustachian tube can be normally passed through the tube during both the active and resolving phases of otitis media [27]. Miura et al. (2002) reported that in six children with cholesteatoma of the middle ear, the pathological findings showed that the lesions mainly occurred in the mastoid cells and the upper recess of the tympanic cavity [28]. Combined with Sade's research, it is suggested that the exudate retained in these blocked areas is mainly due to the obstruction of the internal ventilation drainage channel, rather than poor function of the Eustachian tube. Schachern found in a pathological study of 229 ears and mastoids that 44 ears (19.7%) had complete obstruction of the tympanic antrum by intractable lesions, mainly granulation tissue [29]. Among these 44 ears, the mastoid area of 22 ears had more severe lesions than the middle ear (mainly granulation tissue). Zhang Quan'an et al. found that during the pathological process of otitis media, the degree of mucosal inflammatory lesions in different areas of the middle ear cavity system is not the same, and it is regular that the lesions in the posterior area are significantly more severe than those in the anterior area and the lesions in the ossicular chain area (attic and posterior attic area) are the most severe, which is called the "regional pathological difference phenomenon of otitis media" [30].

When the tympanic membrane is intact, CT examination reveals inflammation in the mastoid, often indicating poor drainage at the second valve near the malleus.

This suggests that the middle ear ventilation system consists of the Eustachian tube (active muscle opening mechanism, mucous clearance mechanism at the tympanic orifice of the tube), tympanic membrane pressure receptors, chemical receptors of the tympanic prominence, second valve (around the malleus), and anterior and posterior isthmuses of the attic, among others. The Eustachian tube is an important active discharge channel in the middle ear ventilation system (equivalent to a small negative pressure suction device), and its lesions are usually temporary (such as colds, air travel, allergic rhinitis, gastroesophageal reflux, etc.). When there is a prolonged lesion, such as enlarged adenoids, nasopharyngeal cancer, congenital anatomical variations, etc., the Eustachian tube cannot actively transport, and the mastoid and attic have no active transport mechanism. After passive transport is obstructed, if it lasts for a long time, biofilms and granulation formation occur, and the lesion becomes irreversible. Even if the Eustachian tube regains function later, the lesions in the mastoid and attic will be left behind and persist, often requiring surgical treatment.

1.8 The Pressure Regulation System of the Middle Ear

The primary function of the middle ear is to transmit sound to the inner ear; hence, maintaining the pressure balance within the middle ear cavity is essential to ensure the normal vibration of the tympanic membrane and the conduction function of the ossicular chain. The regulation of middle ear pressure (MEP) relies not only on the Eustachian tube's regulation but also on the gas exchange between the mastoid mucosa and blood vessels. The mastoid mucosa is a single-layer flat cuboidal epithelium capable of gas exchange, and it has a rich vascular structure beneath the mucosa. The short distance between the mucosal basement layer and the blood vessels facilitates rapid gas exchange. Therefore, the mastoid air cells serve not only as a gas reservoir but also as an important site for gas exchange in the middle ear. The dynamic balance of middle ear pressure depends on the coordinated action of the Eustachian tube's opening and the gas exchange of the mastoid mucosa. Research by Belyea and others has found that some patients who have undergone complete mastoidectomy can maintain ventilation of the remaining middle ear cavity solely through the regulation of the Eustachian tube [31]. However, when there is a significant fluctuation in middle ear pressure, the absence of mastoid air cells as a pressure buffer zone makes it difficult to maintain pressure balance. Gaihede and Ovesen have presented more detailed research results, indicating that when there is a large difference between middle ear pressure and atmospheric pressure, both the opening of the Eustachian tube and the gas exchange of the mastoid mucosa regulate jointly, with the opening of the Eustachian tube playing the primary role [32]. When the difference between middle ear pressure and atmospheric pressure is small, the gas exchange of the mastoid mucosa alone maintains the pressure balance. This view has been debated in the past, and this is a review published in 2019, which still emphasizes the role of the mastoid air cells in maintaining middle ear pressure [33]. The incomplete development of the mastoid air cell system is associated with frequent episodes of otitis media in infants and young children. Most of the mastoid pneumatization process is completed before the age of 5–10.

Another important factor leading to atelectasis of the middle ear and chronic otitis media is the degree of mastoid aeration. The mastoid, an air-containing chamber connected to the middle ear, is often in a state of negative pressure during chronic otitis media. Similar to the middle ear, the mastoid has a pressure-buffering effect, resisting changes in pressure within the middle ear (i.e., Boyle's law). Research by Sade on this closed system of the mastoid has confirmed that the smaller the air cell of the mastoid, the weaker its pressure-buffering capacity, thereby increasing the sensitivity of the tympanic membrane to increased negative pressure in the middle ear [15].

1.9 The Physiological Function of the Nose

The physiological function of the nose is also an essential part of the Eustachian tube system because the air supplied to the Eustachian tube and the middle ear-mastoid must be humidified, warmed, and filtered. A patent nasal cavity is also crucial because nasal obstruction can cause abnormal pharyngeal pressure during swallowing, known as the Toynbee phenomenon.

For a long time, individuals with Eustachian tube dysfunction were considered contraindicated for tympanoplasty, but a large number of foreign studies have shown that there is no difference in the efficacy of tympanoplasty between those with patent and nonpatent Eustachian tubes. This surgical contraindication has long been abolished in Europe and America.

Research indicates that most acute otitis media and secretory otitis media can heal spontaneously without sequelae. Over 80% of purulent otitis media can heal spontaneously, even with a perforated tympanic membrane. This suggests that based on the understanding of the etiology of otitis media, the basic principle of treatment should be antiinfection and elimination of inflammation as the fundamental therapeutic method, while treatment for Eustachian tube dysfunction is difficult to achieve, and clinical practice has also confirmed this. If there is still middle ear effusion after 3 months, tympanotomy or tube placement can be considered. However, repeated incisions and tube placements have the following drawbacks:

(1) They may damage the pressure receptors on the tympanic membrane, which are detrimental to the middle ear ventilation system.
(2) Long-term tube placement can lead to persistent tympanic membrane perforation.
(3) Most tube placements will produce biofilm.
(4) They may induce mold growth.
(5) They can lead to tympanic cavity sclerosis.

A 5-year follow-up study using tympanic membrane tube placement to treat infants with recurrent acute otitis media or chronic secretory otitis media required multiple ventilation tubes, repeated tympanic membrane tube placements, and retraction of the tense part, ultimately leading to underdeveloped mastoids and corresponding reduction in the air cell system.

Study by Post (2001) shown that biofilms within the tympanic membrane ventilation tubes often cause existing infections to persist and be difficult to treat [34]. Jaisingghani et al. (1999) found that out of 150 temporal bones taken from patients with chronic otitis media, 53 (35%) had tympanic membrane sclerosis [35]. Tos and Stangerup performed adenoidectomy on 146 children with bilateral secretory otitis media, placing a tube in the right tympanic membrane and making an incision in the left tympanic membrane [36]. The results showed that 59% of the children had tympanic membrane sclerosis on the right side with the tube while only 13% of the children had the same change in the left ear. Moreover, the tympanic membrane sclerosis secondary to tube placement, with less than 0.5 dB of hearing loss, had little impact.

The main reasons for the nonhealing of tympanic membrane perforations are the following:

(1) The pathogenic bacteria have strong virulence (such as *Pseudomonas aeruginosa*, drug-resistant *Staphylococcus aureus*, *Mycobacterium tuberculosis*, etc.), biofilm formation, and the patient's own immunity is relatively weak. The main pathogens of otitis media are *Streptococcus pneumoniae* and *Haemophilus influenzae*.
(2) Severe mastoid inflammation (irreversible granulation tissue).
(3) Dysfunction of the middle ear ventilation system (Eustachian tube, tympanic antrum, and three valves of the upper middle ear), leading to poor drainage.

There must be mastoiditis with otitis media, just as rhinitis must be accompanied by sinusitis, with only varying degrees of severity. Therefore, otitis media with mild inflammation can often heal spontaneously (more than 80%), and those that cannot heal often have had severe lesions in the mastoid, poor drainage in the mastoid, and a higher possibility of hidden inflammation. Temporal bone CT, even thin-slice CT, often cannot clearly and accurately display the lesions in the mastoid due to the slice thickness being too wide, and the actual situation is often more severe.

Simple tympanic membrane repair (even with Eustachian tube balloon dilation) does not solve the problem of patency and drainage of the mastoid and the upper middle ear. Sometimes, tympanic membrane perforation serves as a natural ventilation tube. If tympanic membrane repair is performed blindly without checking the ventilation of the middle ear, the patient may feel stuffiness in the affected ear after surgery. Ear stuffiness is the second most common discomfort felt by patients after surgery, apart from facial paralysis. There have been many medical disputes in China after simple tympanic membrane repair due to ear stuffiness, which should be taken seriously by colleagues. If hidden inflammation in the mastoid is not removed, it may also affect the healing of the tympanic membrane after surgery and may lead to secondary cholesterol granuloma. Therefore, it is recommended that in addition to traumatic tympanic membrane perforations, all tympanic membrane perforations (i.e., the past simple otitis media), when repairing the tympanic membrane, mastoid exploration should be performed. If the drainage is unobstructed (mastoid injection of saline, by observing the water flow from the tympanic membrane perforation to determine the drainage of the mastoid-tympanic cavity), a simple tympanic membrane repair can be performed directly. If the drainage is not smooth, the treatment principle is as described below for the treatment of middle ear cholesterol granuloma. This treatment principle also solves the past requirement that the ear must be dry for at least 1 month before tympanic membrane repair. Regardless of whether the ear is dry, as long as irreversible lesions are completely removed and drainage is unobstructed, a one-stage tympanic membrane reconstruction can be performed. Moreover, many patients with middle ear and mastoid inflammation cannot dry their ears at all.

At present, there is no particularly accurate test for Eustachian tube function. Acoustic immittance, tympanic pressure graph, drug drops through the perforated tympanic membrane, and Valsalva maneuvers are all indirect examination methods. Elner et al. (1971) found that the positive rate of the Valsalva test in 101 normal adult ears was only 85% [37]. Seventy-nine percent of normal adults had a positive Toynbee test. Wullstein even said that the best way to examine the Eustachian tube is tympanoplasty. Professor Helms found that more than 90% of otitis media and cholesteatoma surgeries found that the Eustachian tube function was basically normal. It is inferred that chronic purulent otitis media and cholesteatoma of the middle ear are due to Eustachian tube dysfunction (the most common reason is adenoid hypertrophy) during childhood, after which the Eustachian tube function recovers, but the middle ear lesion has become an irreversible lesion left behind. Nasopharyngoscopy, laryngoscopy, and otoscopic examination combined with CT examination can roughly determine the site of poor drainage in the middle ear (see the preoperative and postoperative treatment of otoscopic examination). When the Eustachian tube is abnormally open, otoscopic examination should be able to see slight movements of the tympanic membrane synchronized with breathing. The examination must be performed in a sitting position because when lying down (sleeping), due to the absence of venous valves in the head and neck veins, the Eustachian tube is congested, and the abnormally open Eustachian tube usually has no symptoms.

The mastoid air cell system originates from the expansion of the middle ear air-containing cavity from the first pharyngeal pouch, a process that occurs during the development of the temporal bone, leading to varying degrees of mastoid cavity pneumatization. Repeated infections of the middle ear and mastoid restrict the degree of pneumatization of the mastoid air cells. Conversely, the absence of infection is conducive to the full pneumatization of the air cell system. The pneumatization of the middle ear is completed near the age of one. The middle ear and tympanic antrum are the same size as adults in infancy, but the mastoid will continue to grow. Generally, a child's head approaches that of an adult after the age of six. With the development and traction of the sternocleidomastoid muscle, the mastoid also expands. Therefore, a small mastoid suggests that the patient had otitis media in infancy.

In summary, the middle ear ventilation system includes the Eustachian tube (first valve), the area around the malleus (second valve), the anterior and posterior isthmuses of the upper middle ear (third valve), an intact tympanic membrane and its pressure receptors, the chemical (pressure receptor) of the tympanic prominence, the mucociliary clearance system near the Eustachian tube in the tympanic cavity, and the state of nasal function. Combining otoscopic examination with CT examination can roughly determine the condition of the ventilation system:

(1) If the tympanic membrane is intact and there is air in the tympanic cavity, it often indicates that the Eustachian tube function is still acceptable.
(2) The retraction of the tympanic membrane and healing perforation often indicate damage to the pressure receptors on the surface of the tympanic membrane.
(3) Soft tissue shadow in the mastoid indicates dysfunction of the second valve around the malleus.
(4) The inward movement of the manubrium of the malleus, retraction of the tympanic membrane, and retraction of the flaccid part/perforation/cholesteatoma/polyp indicates dysfunction of the third valve in the anterior and posterior isthmuses of the upper middle ear.

At present, there are some easily confused viewpoints in clinical practice. In addition to "secretory otitis media" and "chronic (purulent) otitis media," it is believed that surgery is only indicated when there is a perforation of the tympanic membrane. When there is an obstruction in the middle ear ventilation system, and there are irreversible lesions (granulation tissue, cholesteatoma) in the mastoid or the upper middle ear, even if the tympanic membrane is intact, surgical treatment is necessary, of course, strictly controlling the indications for surgery. Personal opinions are the following:

(1) When the patient complains of obvious ear stuffiness, accompanied by hearing loss, the course of the disease is more than 1 year, and multiple tympanic membrane incisions and tube placements are ineffective.
(2) Under the microscope, the tympanic membrane is seen to be aged and retracted, showing a yellow-brown color (the deeper the color, the longer the course of the disease, the more severe the condition), and the manubrium of the malleus is retracted.
(3) Pure tone audiometry shows conductive deafness.

(4) CT examination shows a large amount of soft tissue shadow in the mastoid and upper middle ear, and surgical treatment should be considered. MRI can help determine the nature of the soft tissue shadow in the mastoid.

References

1. Daly KA, Hunter LL, Giebink GS. Chronic otitis media with effusion[J]. Pediatr Rev. 1999;20(3):85–93.
2. Bluestone CD. Eustachian tube: structure, function, role in otitis media [M]. Translated by Chen Jiaxiang and Chen Shuhua. People's Medical Publishing House; 2009. (Chinese).
3. Post JC, Preston RA, Aul JJ, et al. Molecular analysis of bacterial pathogens in otitis media with effusion[J]. JAMA. 1995;273(20):1598–604.
4. Rayner MG, Zhang Y, Gorry MC, et al. Evidence of bacterial metabolic activity in culture-negative otitis media with effusion[J]. JAMA. 1998;279(4):296–9.
5. Dingman JR, Rayner MG, Mishra S, et al. Correlation between presence of viable bacteria and presence of endotoxin in middle-ear effusions[J]. J Clin Microbiol. 1998;36(11):3417–9.
6. Hall-Stoodley L, Hu FZ, Gieseke A, et al. Direct detection of bacterial biofilms on the middle-ear mucosa of children with chronic otitis media [J]. JAMA. 2006;296:202–11.
7. Gibson WS Jr, Cochran W. Otalgia in infants and children--a manifestation of gastroesophageal reflux[J]. Int J Pediatr Otorhinolaryngol. 1994;28(2-3):213–8.
8. Tasker A, Dettmar PW, Panetti M, et al. Reflux of gastric juice and glue ear in children[J]. Lancet. 2002;359(9305):493.
9. Velepic M, Rozmanic V, Velepic M, et al. Gastroesophageal reflux, allergy and chronic tubo-tympanal disorders in children[J]. Int J Pediatr Otorhinolaryngol. 2000;55(3):187–90.
10. Tasker A, Dettmar PW, Panetti M, et al. Is gastric reflux a cause of otitis media with effusion in children[J]? Laryngoscope. 2002;112(11):1930–4.
11. Poelmans J, Tack J, Feenstra L. Prospective study on the incidence of chronic ear complaints related to gastroesophageal reflux and on the outcome of antireflux therapy[J]. Ann Otol Rhinol Laryngol. 2002;111(10):933–8.
12. Bluestone CD, Klein JO. Otitis media and eustachian tube dysfunction [M]. Philadeiphia: Saunders; 2003. p. 474–685.
13. Trudel M, Laframboise R, Leclerc JE. Musculo-mucous web velum and velopharyngeal dysfunction associated with 8q22.1-22.2 microduplication[J]. Int J Pediatr Otorhinolaryngol. 2018 Jan;104:134–137.
14. Sando I, Takahashi H, Matsune S, et al. Localization of function in the eustachian tube: a hypothesis[J]. Ann Otol Rhinol Laryngol. 1994;103(4 Pt 1):311–4.
15. Sade J. The buffering effect of middle ear negative pressure by retraction of the pars tensa [J]. Am J Otolaryngol. 2000;21:20–3.
16. Honjo I, Hayashi M, Ito S, et al. Pumping and clearance function of the eustachian tube[J]. Am J Otolaryngol. 1985;6(3):241–4.
17. Sadé J, Luntz M. Eustachian tube lumen: comparison between normal and inflamed specimens. Ann Otol Rhinol Laryngol. 1989;98(8 Pt 1):630–4.
18. Zhang Quan'an. Innovative research on theories and clinical practice of otitis media [M]. China Publishing Group; 2013. p. 104. (Chinese).
19. Yang W, Wang R, Sun J. Ultracytochemical observation of secretory cells and surfactant-like lamellar bodies in mucosa of eustachian tube[J]. Zhonghua Er Bi Yan Hou Ke Za Zhi. 1995;30(4):224–6. (Chinese).
20. Fornadley JA, Burns JK. The effect of surfactant on eustachian tube function in a gerbil model of otitis media with effusion[J]. Otolaryngol Head Neck Surg. 1994 ;110(1):110–4.
21. Nemechek AJ, Pahlavan N, Cote DN. Nebulized surfactant for experimentally induced otitis media with effusion[J]. Otolaryngol Head Neck Surg. 1997;117(5):475–9.
22. Zhu ZH, Shan YJ, Han Y, et al. Pathological study of otitis media with effusion after treatment with intranasal pulmonary surfactant. Laryngoscope. 2013;123(12):3148–55.
23. White DR, Heavner SB, Hardy SM, et al. Gastroesophageal reflux and eustachian tube dysfunction in an animal model[J]. Laryngoscope. 2002;112(6):955–61.
24. Eden AR, Ganon PI. Neural control of middle-ear aeration [J]. Arch Otolaryngol Head Neck Surg. 1987;113:133–7.
25. Shupak A, Tabari R, Swarts JD, et al. Effects of middle-ear oxygen and carbon dioxide tensions on Eustachian tube ventilatory function [J]. Laryngoscope. 1996;106:221–4.
26. Zhang Quan'an, Wang Li, Wei Junrong. Obstruction of internal ventilation and drainage in the pathological process of otitis media [J]. J Xi'an Med Univ. 1999;2:536–9. (Chinese)
27. Takahashi H, Hayashi M, Stato H, et al. Primary deficits in eustachian tube function in patients with otitis media with effusion [J]. Arch Otolaryngol Head Neck Surg. 1989;115(5):581–4.
28. Miura M, Sando I, Orita Y, et al. Histopathologic study of the temporal bones and Eustachian tubes of children with cholesterol granuloma[J]. Ann Otol Rhinol Laryngol. 2002;111(7 Pt 1):609–15.
29. Schachern PA, Paparella MM, Sano S, et al. A histopathological study of the relationship between

otitis media and mastoiditis [J]. Laryngoscope. 1991;101(10):1050–5.
30. Zhang Quan'an, Zhang Xiaotong, Zhang Qing, et al. A study on the regional pathological differences and clinical significance in otitis media [J]. Chin J Otorhinolaryngol. 2004;39(9):534–7. (Chinese)
31. Belyea J, Wickens B, Bance M. Middle ear ventilation status postoperatively after translabyrinthine resection of vestibular schwannoma with mastoid obliteration and Eustachian tube occlusion: is the Eustachian tube enough to ventilate the middle ear without the mastoid air cell system[J]? J Otolaryngol Head Neck Surg. 2016;45(1):44.
32. Gaihede M, Ovesen T. Precision of tympanometric measurements[J]. J Speech Lang Hear Res. 1997;40(1):215–22.
33. Lin Qiongping et al. Research progress on the excretory and absorptive functions of the middle ear cavity mucosa. Int J Otorhinolaryngol Head Neck Surg. 2019;43(4).
34. Post JC. Direct evidence of bacterial biofilms in otitis media[J]. Laryngoscope. 2001;111(12):2083–94.
35. Jaisinghani VJ, Paparella MM, Schachern PA, et al. Tympanic membrane/middle ear pathologic correlates in chronic otitis media[J]. Laryngoscope. 1999;109(5):712–6.
36. Tos M, Stangerup SE. Hearing loss in tympanosclerosis caused by grommets [J]. Arch Otolaryngol Head Neck Surg. 1989;115:931–5.
37. Elner A, Ingelstedt S, Ivarsson A. The normal function of the eustachian tube. A study of 102 cases[J]. Acta Otolaryngol. 1971;72(5):320–8.

Perioperative Management of Suppurative Otitis Media

2

Tongxiang Diao, Qingyang Shi, and Lisheng Yu

Chronic suppurative otitis media (CSOM) is a potentially life-threatening condition, frequently encountered in geriatric patients with a protracted history of the disease, often presenting with compromised systemic health rendering them intolerant to surgical intervention. In such precarious clinical scenarios, management becomes highly challenging. It is therefore imperative to counsel patients on the necessity of early surgical treatment. This measure serves dual purposes: first, it aims to prevent severe intracranial and extracranial complications, thereby ensuring patient safety; secondly, it contributes to improved quality of life and may lead to a reduction in healthcare costs. Physicians bear the responsibility of elucidating the risks and benefits of surgery, including explaining that the hazards associated with the illness necessitate prompt action. They must discuss the likelihoods of various outcomes, such as an approximate 80% rate of hearing improvement, a one-third chance of tinnitus amelioration, and a recurrence rate for cholesteatoma below 10%. However, while medical professionals can strongly advise on the surgical option, they do not hold the ultimate decision-making authority unless the patient's life is immediately endangered, in which case emergency measures may be indicated. The informed consent process encompasses these aspects of potential risks, benefits, symptom improvements, and probabilities of recurrence.

2.1 Preoperative Consultation

Preoperative consultation considerations include the following:

(1) Emphasize that chronic suppurative otitis media and cholesteatoma are potentially life-threatening conditions; hence the paramount principle of surgery is preservation of life through comprehensive eradication of pathological changes to avert fatal complications. It is noteworthy that while patients frequently inquire about surgical risks, it is often the inherent dangers of the disease rather than the surgery itself that pose significant threats, akin to the existence of hazards on the street, which does not deter people from venturing out.
(2) A steadfast commitment to safeguarding vital functional structures, such as the facial nerve, major vasculature (internal carotid artery, jugular bulb, sigmoid sinus), and

T. Diao · Q. Shi · L. Yu (✉)
Department of Otorhinolaryngology, Head and Neck Surgery, People's Hospital, Peking University, Beijing, China
e-mail: 1710301204@pku.edu.cn

L. Yu (ed.), *Progress in Postauricular Administration*, Experts' Perspectives on Medical Advances,
https://doi.org/10.1007/978-981-95-5102-6_2

meninges, is imperative during the surgical intervention.

(3) Efforts must be exerted to protect (or reconstruct) auditory transmission mechanisms, with even the world's most accomplished otologic surgeons achieving an approximate 80% efficacy rate in improving hearing postoperatively.
(4) Stress the indispensable nature of postoperative follow-up assessments, as they are critical for monitoring recovery and detecting potential issues early.
(5) Acknowledge the possibility of reoperation under special circumstances, exemplified by the need for a "second-look" procedure in cases of congenital cholesteatoma.

In instances where patients harbor unrealistic expectations, such as the resolution of tinnitus through this surgery, provide thorough elucidation and informed consent. If, despite counseling, the patient insists on pursuing unrealistic goals, abstaining from surgery may be considered. As articulated by the renowned surgical professor Atul Gawande from Harvard Medical School in his book *The Checklist Manifesto*, physicians perennially grapple with the paradoxical challenge of navigating uncertainty while striving for optimal outcomes.

In Germany, preoperative consultations are typically conducted in an outpatient setting and are facilitated by the attending physician assigned to the specialist's clinic. Patients with questions or concerns have the opportunity to directly engage in dialogue with the operating surgeon themselves. For each medical condition, standardized preoperative consultation forms are utilized to ensure comprehensive coverage and prevent any omissions. The conduct of a preoperative conversation is indeed an art form; when executed effectively, it can forestall numerous unnecessary disputes. If, following every such consultation, patients consistently opt against surgery, it could be argued that the consulting physician has not fully succeeded in their role. Nevertheless, it is imperative that physicians do not exaggerate their abilities or therapeutic outcomes merely to persuade patients towards undergoing surgery.

2.2 Preoperative Examination Preparation

2.2.1 Medical History Acquisition

Given that many patients have a disease onset during childhood, providing an accurate history of the condition can be challenging. Key inquiry points include the following:

① Principal symptoms of chronic suppurative otitis media, such as otorrhea, hearing loss, tinnitus, and aural fullness, relevant treatment history, and inclusive of surgical interventions.
② The presence and status of intracranial and extracranial complications, including symptoms like vertigo, facial paralysis, periauricular swelling, headaches, and high fever.
③ Distinguishing diagnoses, such as tuberculous otitis media, HIV/AIDS, otosclerosis, and tumors involving the facial nerve.
④ Inquiry into systemic diseases and medications that may impact surgery, with menstrual history being queried for female patients. Elderly patients and those with systemic conditions must undergo preoperative evaluations and treatments at the anesthesia department and relevant specialties accordingly.
⑤ Understanding the patient's expectations regarding treatment outcomes.

2.2.2 Otoscopic examination

It's paramount, its significance far outweighing the information provided by tympanometry. Otologists should cultivate a sound habit of meticulously clearing earwax, secretions, and crusts from the ear canal to discern every detail of the ear canal and tympanic membrane. Microscopes and/or endoscopes may be employed when necessary. An inward displacement of the malleus handle or tympanic annulus often suggests poor drainage in the attic space. Chronic congestion and edema in the tympanic annulus or the bony part of the external auditory canal frequently indicate gastroesophageal reflux and/or occult otitis media with effusion. Pallor and edema of the tympanic annulus are often indicative of allergic otitis media secondary to allergic rhinitis. A polyp originating from the base of the tympanic annulus is termed a signal polyp, commonly suggesting cholesteatoma in the attic. A yellow discoloration behind the tympanic membrane often suggests inadequate drainage of the malleus and the presence of a cholesterol granuloma within the mastoid. Suggestive white opacity behind the tympanic membrane necessitates exclusion of congenital cholesteatoma. In cases with prior surgical history, recurrence of cholesteatoma should be considered. If the posterior aspect of the tympanic membrane appears reddened, CT scan results should be integrated. Absence of a mass lesion should prompt consideration of Schwartze's sign (otosclerosis), while the presence of a mass lesion might suggest a glomus tympanicum tumor. Blue tympanic membranes are most commonly associated with cholesteatomas, blood accumulation (posttrauma, hematological disorders, etc.), or a high-riding jugular bulb. Granulation tissue found on the floor of the external auditory canal is indicative of malignant external otitis, that is, skull base osteomyelitis [1].

2.2.3 Audiological Assessment

Patients with conductive or mixed hearing loss often speak at a lower volume, as they can hear their own voice well through bone conduction and are less affected by ambient noise interference. Consequently, in noisy environments, their speech may sound quieter to normal-hearing individuals who tend to raise their voices to compensate for the noise. Therefore, patients presenting with normal or reduced speaking volume during consultation have a higher likelihood of benefiting from tympanoplasty for hearing improvement. Conversely, those who habitually speak loudly typically indicate severe or profound sensorineural hearing loss, rendering them less likely to experience improved hearing from tympanoplasty. Electroacoustic testing (audiometry) can provide a preliminary assessment of ossicular chain status through the audiogram. In cases where the tympanic membrane is intact (or patched following perforation), an air-bone gap (ABG) < 20 dB suggests conditions such as otitis media with effusion or gastric acid reflux. An ABG of 20–40 dB indicates restricted ossicular mobility, often due to mucosal edema or granulation tissue near the ossicular chain. An ABG of 50–60 dB suggests ossicular discontinuity. It is noteworthy that not only middle ear pathologies present with conductive hearing loss; certain inner ear disorders can also exhibit ABGs (mixed conductive-sensorineural hearing loss), including large vestibular aqueduct syndrome, Meniere's disease, some cases of sudden sensorineural hearing loss, superior semicircular canal dehiscence syndrome, and X-linked stapes gusher syndrome, among others. Additionally, certain middle ear pathologies can cause sensorineural hearing loss, like the effects of otitis media on the inner ear (specific types include allergic otitis media and tuberculous otitis media), gastric acid reflux-related otosclerosis, osteogenesis imperfecta, Paget's disease, and middle ear tumors affecting inner ear function. A proficient otologist should master tuning fork tests since, even when combined with precise pure tone audiometry, these tests can be superior in differentiating sensorineural from conductive hearing loss based on case history.

2.2.4 Assessing Eustachian Tube Function

(Refer to Otitis Media and the Middle Ear Ventilation System)

2.2.5 Fiber Nasopharyngoscopy and Laryngoscopy

These examinations are crucial for excluding nasopharyngeal space-occupying lesions (such as nasopharyngeal carcinoma), chronic rhinosinusitis, adenoid hypertrophy (residual), allergic rhinitis, and gastric acid reflux. They significantly guide perioperative treatment strategies, including medication administration.

2.2.6 Imaging Studies

Generally, CT scans hold paramount importance. They play a critical role in determining the extent, nature of the lesion, surgical incision, and approach. CTs are also instrumental in assessing disease progression. Repeated infections in the middle ear and mastoid hinder pneumatization, whereas absence of infection promotes optimal pneumatization. Middle ear aeration completes around 1 year of age, with the middle ear and mesotympanum attaining adult size during infancy while the mastoid continues to grow. The mastoid expands with the development of the sternocleidomastoid muscle; hence small mastoids suggest a history of middle ear infection during early childhood. In select cases, MRI might be necessary to rule out glomus jugulare tumors, pontomedullary junction lesions, endolymphatic sac tumors, and petrous apex pathologies. CT scans primarily focus on mastoid size, pneumatization, distance between the sigmoid sinus and external auditory canal, tegmen tympani position, location of the facial nerve, presence of bony coverage, and the surrounding ossicular environment. Diagnosis of labyrinthitis relies heavily on characteristic clinical presentations, complemented by gadolinium-enhanced T1-weighted MRI showing infectious changes in the labyrinth (Dobben GD et al., 2000). Preoperative image interpretation is crucial. Prof. Draf has an exemplary practice of joint radiology-otorhinolaryngology film reading sessions between 7 and 8 AM, which benefits both specialties. To prevent errors in surgical side identification, it is recommended that surgeons review imaging studies once again before surgery.

2.2.7 Bacterial Cultures

Preoperative secretion cultures guide surgery and antibiotic selection. For virulent bacteria like *Pseudomonas aeruginosa*, *Mycobacterium tuberculosis*, and drug-resistant *Staphylococcus aureus*, open surgical techniques are preferred.

2.2.8 General Examination Preparation

Beyond routine preoperative preparations, particular attention must be given to systemic diseases that could impact surgery. High-risk patients should undergo preoperative evaluation by the anesthesia department to determine their suitability for surgery. Most surgeries in otolaryngology-head and neck surgery, except for emergencies related to bleeding, foreign bodies, respiratory distress, life-threatening cancers, or intracranial tumors, are elective procedures and should be meticulously prepared for. Perioperative risks are often associated with systemic health issues rather than the surgery itself.

2.3 Preoperative and Postoperative Medication Usage

The application of 3% hydrogen peroxide and ofloxacin otic drops are both common local therapeutic modalities in otology. My mentor, Professor Helms, was notably surprised by our use of hydrogen peroxide eardrops and sternly cautioned that such a practice is fraught with peril. The reason for this concern lies in the potential presence of congenital (e.g., malformations) or acquired (inflammatory processes, cholesteatoma erosion) pathways connecting the middle ear to the intracranial space, which may be unrecognized. A case during a consultation vividly underscored this danger: a patient with chronic suppurative otitis media presented with a small tympanic membrane perforation and purulent discharge. The attending physician administered 3% hydrogen peroxide into the middle ear cavity via the perforation using a syringe, resulting in an immediate collapse of the patient who experienced convulsions and unconsciousness. Despite successful resuscitation, the patient sustained profound unilateral deafness and blindness in the ipsilateral eye. This adverse outcome aligns with Professor Helms' warning regarding the existence of a potential communication between the middle ear and the cranial cavity, wherein hydrogen peroxide ingress could lead to increased intracranial pressure and, in severe cases, brain herniation with fatal consequences. Consequently, extreme caution must be exercised when employing hydrogen peroxide in patients with chronic suppurative otitis media or cholesteatoma. Additionally, there is a compelling argument against the routine use of topical antibiotics in such scenarios. Given the presence of pus, granulation tissue, cholesteatoma, and sclerotic foci within the middle ear and mastoid cavities, local antibiotic administration is unlikely to reach all areas effectively, thereby increasing the risk of fostering bacterial resistance and concomitant fungal infections.

2.4 Postoperative Follow-Up and Dressing Changes

(1) Sutures are typically removed 1 week post-surgery. When removing sutures from an intracanalicular incision, it is essential to exercise caution as overly tight packing may lead to wound dehiscence upon suture removal. Therefore, 2 days prior to the scheduled suture removal, it is advisable to loosen and partially remove gauze strips packed at the external auditory canal entrance to alleviate tension and prevent wound rupture during the suture extraction process.

(2) The packing of iodoform gauze within the surgical cavity should be removed approximately 2–3 weeks after surgery. Following mastoidectomy, three types of tissue growth occur within the cavity: epithelium, mucosa, and granulation tissue. It is generally observed that respiratory mucosal epithelium has a faster turnover rate than skin epithelium. Furthermore, under conditions such as high-dose radiation therapy or antitumor drug use, mucosal reactions tend to manifest earlier and more severely compared to skin reactions, reflecting their differing rates of renewal. Epithelial regeneration is the slowest, while granulation tissue proliferates most rapidly. In early cases of chronic otitis media surgery, removal of the surgical cavity packing within 1 week can result in complicated postoperative care, often necessitating hospitalization for dressing changes for about a month. Notably, Professor Helms's mentor, the renowned otologist Plester, once encountered a patient who inadvertently missed their follow-up appointment, returning only 3 weeks later. Surprisingly, the outcome was excellent; upon removal of the iodoform packing, the ear quickly achieved a dry state, suggesting that maintaining some pressure within the surgical cavity can effectively suppress granulation tissue growth. Consequently, it is advisable to delay the removal of iodoform-packed gauze within the ear canal as much as possible. During each dressing change, closely monitor the color of the gauze—yellowing indicates that it can remain for an extended period, whereas a white coloration due to increased secretion suggests that the gauze should be removed. If the gauze must be extracted within 2 weeks postsurgery, it can be repacked with iodoform gauze. In individual cases where patients exhibit iodoform allergy, antibiotic and steroid ointment-infused gauze can be used for packing, but these must be changed every 3–5 days. For patients with congenital atresia of the external auditory canal, the duration of iodoform gauze packing may need to be extended up to 5–6 weeks.

(3) Upon the initial removal of iodoform gauze, refrain from disturbing the innermost absorbent cotton; allow it to remain in place for an additional week or so, which may abbreviate the time to a dry ear canal. After extracting all packing materials, instruct patients to maintain adequate ventilation within the surgical cavity and avoid obstructing the external auditory canal with cotton balls.

(4) Postoperative follow-up and dressing changes are critically important, requiring

meticulous cleaning of any secretions within the surgical cavity each time. Smaller granulations should be excised, with their bases cauterized using 50% trichloroacetic acid.

(5) The primary failure rate of the initial radical mastoidectomy ranges from 3% to 26%. Blockage of the attic opening is among the leading causes of failure. In cases where the ear does not attain a dry state postoperatively, factors beyond the surgery itself (such as inadequate removal of air cells, excessively high facial ridge, residual disease, poor drainage, and untimely dressing changes resulting in granulation proliferation) have been identified, including allergies, gastroesophageal reflux (GERD), and migraines. GERD, particularly acidic gases, initially affects the upper part of the middle ear via the Eustachian tube, often presenting with congestion and edema at the tympanic membrane's annulus, increased secretion. Migraines, characterized by excessive trigeminal nerve excitement and vasodilation, can also contribute to excessive secretion in the surgical cavity, thus preventing a dry ear. Targeted treatments are necessary; for example, if there is substantial exposed bone in the cavity, use ear-specific absorbent cotton, applying corticosteroid nasal sprays twice daily.

(6) When encountering wound infection or dehiscence after suture removal in the postauricular area, thoroughly disinfect the site using povidone-iodine and alcohol before scraping away all necrotic tissue with a curette. Subsequently, clean the wound again with povidone-iodine and alcohol, and then pack the entire wound with granulated sugar, repeating this method for several days. Due to its high concentration and potent bactericidal properties, sugar promotes granulation tissue growth, and after several days, no further secretion should occur, allowing for direct suturing. This similar dressing technique can be applied to pharyngeal leaks and infected preauricular fistulas.

(7) A first-line antibiotic, such as a cephalosporin, can be administered 1 week postsurgery. Thereafter, for minimal secretion in the surgical cavity, consider a second-line antibiotic like clarithromycin for 1–2 weeks. Depending on the situation, antireflux medication, mucolytics, and other medications might be prescribed. If there is mucosal edema within the surgical cavity, a corticosteroid nasal spray can be used twice daily.

(8) For postoperative narrowing of the external auditory canal, consider using high-expansion nasal sponge for dilation for 1–2 weeks, changing weekly. Apply corticosteroid nasal spray twice daily to prevent drying. Following dilation, a silicone ear mold can be custom-made by a hearing aid company, ensuring that the vent hole is made large enough to guarantee proper ventilation of the external auditory canal. However, long-term usage of high-expansion sponges is not recommended.

(9) Historically, Valsalva maneuver (pinching the nose while blowing) was advised post-surgery to facilitate early aeration of the middle ear. Recent findings suggest that patients with chronic suppurative otitis media and cholesteatoma have a high likelihood of concurrent GERD. Therefore, it is now recommended to substitute the Tonby maneuver (holding water in the mouth and swallowing while pinching the nose) to mitigate the impact of GERD on Eustachian tube function. As needed, antacid medication can be taken orally.

2.5 Postoperative Symptom Explanations and Management

2.5.1 Impaired Hearing

Postoperative hearing impairment can stem from various factors. When the bone-air conduction gap is within 30 dB, conservative management may be pursued, involving oral administration of mucolytic agents and acid suppressants, among other medications. If such interventions prove ineffective, patients can be fitted with hearing aids. In cases where the bone-air conduction gap exceeds 40 dB, a reoperation may be considered, or osseointegrated bone conduction implants could be an option. Although secondary surgery for hearing reconstruction significantly increases the likelihood of postoperative hearing improvement, it is recommended that efforts to reconstruct hearing are maximized during the initial surgical intervention, as this approach also carries an approximate 80% probability of successful auditory enhancement. The primary goal of the first surgery is often to alleviate life-threatening conditions, which most patients readily accept. However, when the aim of a second surgery is solely to improve hearing, even with an 80% success rate, it concurrently implies that approximately 20% of patients might experience unsatisfactory hearing recovery. Given the current medical landscape, it is advisable to minimize interventions with uncertain outcomes. For mild to moderate sensorineural hearing loss, conservative treatments including the use of medications like betahistine and ginkgo leaf extracts, in conjunction with hearing aids, may be appropriate. For severe to profound hearing loss, cochlear implantation should be contemplated.

2.5.2 Tinnitus

Studies by Helms et al. have shown that following middle ear surgery, one-third of patients experience reduced or eliminated tinnitus, one-third remain unchanged, and one-third report worsening symptoms. The causal relationship between tinnitus and middle ear surgery is complex; thus it cannot be guaranteed to patients that tinnitus will improve through surgical intervention. Detailed knowledge about tinnitus can be found in the chapter titled "Tinnitus." In otosclerosis surgery, approximately 90% of patients report a decrease or disappearance of tinnitus. The mechanism underlying this improvement may be attributed to the masking effect of excessively loud internal sounds. A German study once placed 20 university students with normal hearing and no history of tinnitus in a soundproof room for 2 h; afterward, all participants reported experiencing tinnitus during the isolation period. Essentially, every healthy individual has tinnitus, but environmental noise masks these internal sounds, rendering them imperceptible. For conductive hearing loss patients, the decreased hearing leads to the disappearance of this masking effect, causing self-perceived tinnitus. In some migraine sufferers, the mechanism of tinnitus resembles auditory hypersensitivity, where increased auditory sensitivity gives rise to the perception of tinnitus.

2.5.3 Ear Fullness

Eustachian tube dysfunction, inner ear disorders (such as endolymphatic hydrops), and migraines are among the conditions that can cause a feeling of fullness in the ear. The temporal characteristics of the symptoms can aid in differentiation. For instance, Eustachian tube dysfunction, often caused by gastroesophageal reflux, tends to alleviate in a supine position, resulting in milder symptoms upon waking, which then gradually worsen throughout the day. Conversely, in cases of endolymphatic hydrops, the condition exacerbates upon lying down due to worsened venous return, leading to more severe symptoms in the morning. Moreover, preoperative retraction pockets in the tympanic membrane, tight apposition of the malleus handle against the promontory, and poor attic and mastoid drainage without removal of the incus during surgery can also lead to postoperative ear fullness sensations.

2.5.4 Facial Paralysis

Facial paralysis can be categorized as immediate or delayed onset. Local anesthetics, direct exposure of the facial nerve, and excessive packing pressure can occasionally induce immediate facial paralysis, albeit typically mild and transient. Immediate onset signifies intraoperative injury, with mild damage often resulting from overstretching of the chorda tympani, dissection around granulation tissue covering the facial nerve, stimulation during cholesteatoma removal, or improper use of the drill, as well as excessive energy delivered by bipolar electrocautery. Mild cases can be managed conservatively, while those with severe damage exceeding 90% necessitate facial nerve repair surgery.

2.5.5 Dizziness

Postoperative dizziness after middle ear surgery can stem from various causes, each requiring specific identification and management. Potential reasons include the following:

(1) Dislodged otoconia due to prolonged head positioning and drill usage, leading to benign paroxysmal positional vertigo (BPPV). Diagnosis can be confirmed with positional testing, followed by canalith repositioning maneuvers.
(2) Overly tight packing of the external ear canal irritating the vestibular system and simple relief of packing suffices.
(3) Hydrops in the utricle or saccule, for which betahistine may be prescribed.
(4) Presence of a fistula or prolonged irrigation with cold saline during surgery.
(5) Preexisting vestibular diseases such as vestibular migraine or Meniere's disease.

2.5.6 Symptoms Unexplained by Current Diagnostic Tools

A case was encountered where a patient with chronic otitis media experienced severe ear pain postoperatively. Upon examination, the surgical cavity was dry, and a follow-up CT scan appeared normal. When existing diagnostic tests and medical knowledge fail to provide a plausible explanation, mental health issues must be considered. This particular patient was later diagnosed with schizophrenia.

Reference

1. Snow JB Jr, Ashley Wackym P. Ballenger's otorhinolaryngology—head and neck surgery [M]. Li Daqing. Beijing: People's Medical Publishing House; 2012. p. 195.

3 Principles of Surgery for Chronic Suppurative Otitis Media

Tongxiang Diao, Jiahua Luo, and Lisheng Yu

3.1 On the Selection of Surgical Incisions and Approaches

The surgical incision and approach are determined based on factors such as age, mastoid pneumatization, extent of the lesion, and the ability to return for follow-up.

(1) For simple tympanic membrane repair, if the anterior edge of the tympanic membrane perforation can be clearly seen from within the ear canal, an endaural incision can generally be used. Sometimes, due to the forward bulging of the anterior wall of the external auditory canal or the narrowing of the external auditory canal, the anterior edge of the tympanic membrane perforation cannot be seen from within the ear canal. In such cases, a postauricular incision is recommended.

(2) For pediatric and young patients: Preferably perform canal wall down procedures, especially for children. Due to the inconvenience of postoperative dressing changes, it is advisable to use canal wall down techniques. For elderly patients, prioritize canal wall up styles, as these patients often have poor Eustachian tube function, a longer disease course, and poorly developed or sclerotic mastoids.

(3) Mastoid pneumatization: Poor pneumatization, anterior displacement of the sigmoid sinus (distance between the sigmoid sinus and the posterior wall of the external auditory canal is less than 1.5 cm), sclerotic mastoid, and low-lying tegmen typically require an endaural incision and canal wall up technique. If pneumatization is good or even excessive, a postauricular incision and intact canal wall technique are used. If the inflammation is severe and the intact canal wall technique cannot be applied, after thoroughly removing the lesions, the mastoid cavity should be narrowed using materials such as cartilage, bone powder, or flaps.

(4) When complications are present, canal wall up surgery is often utilized. In cases of severe bacterial infections, such as *Pseudomonas aeruginosa*, *Mycobacterium tuberculosis*, or drug-resistant *Staphylococcus aureus*, canal wall up surgery is also preferred whenever possible.

(5) For recurrent surgeries and second-stage surgeries aimed at improving hearing, they should be performed by experienced and senior doctors. For recurrent cholesteatoma surgeries, an open surgical approach should be adopted whenever possible.

T. Diao · J. Luo · L. Yu (✉)
Department of Otorhinolaryngology, Head and Neck Surgery, People's Hospital, Peking University, Beijing, China

L. Yu (ed.), *Progress in Postauricular Administration*, Experts' Perspectives on Medical Advances,
https://doi.org/10.1007/978-981-95-5102-6_3

3.2 Surgical Techniques

(1) Position: For ENT surgery, it is best to elevate the upper body by 15° to reduce intraoperative bleeding. The head should be extended along with the shoulders to avoid obstructing the surgeon's operation. Tilt the head 45° so that the surgeon can easily see the external auditory canal and tympanic membrane while seated.

(2) Disinfection: Iodine has ototoxicity and may cause complete deafness in some patients. Therefore, iodine tincture or iodophor should not be directly used to soak the external auditory canal during disinfection. Instead, a cotton ball should be placed at the entrance of the external auditory canal and moistened. The deeper part of the external auditory canal should be disinfected with an alcohol-soaked cotton ball. When the eardrum is intact, the deeper part of the external auditory canal is sterile. For purulent otitis media or cholesteatoma, soaking with iodophor cannot achieve thorough sterilization. The function of iodine is to sterilize, and alcohol is to inhibit bacteria. Gelatin sponge also has ototoxicity, and if placed in the tympanic cavity, it may stimulate granulation growth, so it is not recommended for use.

(3) Anesthesia: Even under general anesthesia, it is recommended to perform local block anesthesia. For adult patients, use 10 ml of 2% lidocaine with 8–10 drops of epinephrine. This can reduce intraoperative bleeding, decrease the amount of general anesthetics needed during surgery, and result in less postoperative pain for the patient. For pediatric patients, use 10 ml of 1% lidocaine with 3–6 drops of epinephrine. Longer-acting medications, such as bupivacaine, can also be used, especially for pediatric patients, as it significantly reduces postoperative pain.

(4) Equipment preparation: surgical microscope, electric drill, bipolar coagulator, electric knife, ear microsurgery instruments, etc. For German ear surgery, usually two scalpel handles are prepared, one with a size 10 blade and one with a size 15 blade. A larger blade is used for the incision, and a smaller blade is used when cutting the skin flap of the external auditory canal.

3.3 Precautions and Procedures for Surgeries with Different Incisions

3.3.1 Intraauricular incision

The first cut should reach the bone surface, and when cutting outward, it should be shallower to ensure it cuts on the outer side of the temporalis muscle, as there is a blood vessel inside the temporalis muscle. Cutting too deep will cause bleeding.

If there is a perforation in the eardrum, freshening the edges is necessary first. Before making an incision in the ear canal skin flap, use a hook knife to circumcise parts of the perforation edges of the eardrum to create fresh edges. Only the anterior and inferior parts need to be cut, and then the cut edges of the eardrum can be clamped with micro forceps. If the ear canal skin flap is incised first, the eardrum will become soft, making it difficult to create fresh edges. Calcified plaques must also be removed, as they can block new blood vessels and affect the healing of the repair material. Therefore, what initially appears to be a small perforation may become a large one after freshening the edges and removing the calcified plaques.

Then create a serpentine flap of the external auditory canal. If only a tympanum exploration is performed, the serpentine flap can be made smaller, starting from the 1 to 2 o'clock position, making it easier to handle the smaller rolled-up flap. If the superior tympanum and mastoid are also to be opened, the flap should be made larger, extending up to the 12 o'clock position. Use a spatula to lift the serpentine flap and push it forward until reaching the annulus, and then use a hook knife to open and expose the tympanic cavity. The external auditory canal plays an important role in transmitting sound to the eardrum. The acute angle formed by the eardrum and the anterior part of the external auditory canal helps in creating significant sound pressure changes in different regions of the eardrum in the high-frequency range. Therefore, it is best not to lift the anterior wall flap of the external auditory canal during surgery.

Use a bone curette to remove part of the posterior wall of the external auditory canal until the long process of the incus and the stapes footplate are visible. When using the bone curette to scrape the posterior wall of the external auditory canal, be sure to apply an outward force to prevent slipping inward. Prepare a small bowl with saline solution for cleaning the curette.

If canal wall up mastoidectomy is required and the bone is too hard, it can be very difficult to remove the posterior wall of the external auditory canal using a curette. In such cases, a drill is needed. In Germany, the common practice is to directly remove the skin flap of the external auditory canal and preserve it in 0.9% saline gauze and then place it back in its original position after the procedure. This approach provides better exposure and avoids the risk of the skin flap being torn by the drill. We have now made some improvements: by using a small cotton ball to press down the skin flap and carefully coordinating the procedure, the skin flap can be prevented from tearing. At the end of the surgery, the skin flap is placed back in its original position. The closer to the external auditory canal opening, the thicker the skin flap. Excessively thick subcutaneous tissue can be trimmed with ophthalmic scissors to thin the flap.

To fully assess the condition of the ossicular chain, it is necessary to clearly see the incudostapedial joint, the base of the stapes, and the anterior ligament of the malleus located at the anterosuperior part of the malleus.

An enlarged intraaural incision can reveal the function of the malleus, particularly the impact of the anterior side of the malleus handle and the short process of the malleus on its movement. The anterior ligament of the malleus determines the movement of the malleus handle and the malleus. Therefore, to observe the movement of the malleus, it is necessary to see above the short process of the malleus and the anterior ligament of the malleus. Using a diamond drill bit, the bone in front is ground away until the annulus tympanicus is clearly visible. Malleus fixation is sometimes partial. The reason for poor hearing outcomes in 30% of stapedectomy surgeries is malleus movement impairment. If the malleus head is fixed, it needs to be severed to improve malleus movement. If the malleus handle remains, it can be directly connected to the stapes, and postoperative air-bone gap can be within 20 dB. If the malleus, incus, and the upper structure of the stapes are missing, the postoperative air-bone gap may be over 30 dB.

The sequence of ossicular chain exploration is as followed: First, use a hook knife or micro hook to gently lift the handle of the malleus upward and outward, and observe the movement of the long process of the incus. Then, gently pull the long process of the incus inward and upward, and observe the movement of the stapes. Finally, move the two crura of the stapes and observe the activity of the stapes footplate to determine which part has a problem.

When examining the movement of the ossicular chain, attention should be paid to checking the condition of the ligaments with a probe. Sclerosis and fixation of the anterior malleal ligament can lead to significant hearing loss. Studies using laser Doppler interferometry have found that artificial fixation of the anterior malleal ligament can cause 0–12 dB of conductive hearing loss. It is estimated that 38% of patients with residual conductive hearing loss after stapedectomy have fixation of the anterior malleal ligament. The fixed ligament can be severed using a hook knife or laser, which can enlarge the space above the anterior process of the malleus. The treatment of tensor tympani muscle sclerosis is not difficult; it can be severed with a hook knife without affecting the vibration of the tympanic membrane. After severing the tensor tympani muscle, it is often possible to release the contact between the malleus handle and the promontory.

The diagnosis of idiopathic malleus fixation requires observation of movement under a Siegle otoscope. There are two methods to address this issue. The more time-consuming but physiologically preferable method is to remove the bony bridge between the superior tympanic cavity and the malleus head through a mastoidectomy. Care should be taken to avoid direct contact with the malleus when using a drill. First, thin the lateral wall of the superior tympanic cavity at a low drill speed, and it is best to remove the bony bridge using a bone curette or laser to avoid noise-induced damage to the inner ear, as contact with the malleus by the drill can produce noise levels exceeding 120 dB.

3.3.2 Postauricular incision

The skin incision varies depending on the type of surgery. For middle ear infections or Ménière's disease, the incision should be closer to the auricular cartilage, generally 0.5–1 cm behind the postauricular groove. For cochlear implant surgery or acoustic neuroma surgery, the incision should be slightly further back, about 1–1.5 cm. In newborns and infants, the facial nerve runs superficially and is susceptible to injury during forceps-assisted delivery and mastoid surgery, requiring special attention.

The reason for the T-shaped incision of the subperiosteal flap is to avoid damaging the vessels from the front (superficial temporal artery and vein), below (posterior auricular vessels), and the occipital region. This way, the incision is not the same as the flap incision, which to some extent can reduce wound healing difficulties caused by vascular injury. Similarly, different surgeries have different requirements. For example, in Meniere's disease or when preparing for a wall-down tympanoplasty, the focus of the surgery is near the sinus tympani, so the lower incision should not be too low as the mastoid tip is not the focus. However, for facial nerve decompression, extensive chronic suppurative otitis media, cholesteatoma, and other conditions, the lower incision needs to be larger. When making the incision, it is not entirely a sharp dissection; often the blade is used to press open the subcutaneous tissue, which can prevent errors in the dissection layers and ensure adequate hemostasis.

The tegmen tympani in children is often low, so when opening the mastoid, it is essential to start from the bottom and work upward to avoid damaging the dura mater. After opening the mastoid and gradually removing the mastoid bone, the mastoid antrum is usually visible. The mastoid antrum is generally located at the upper inner part of the mastoid region. The opening of the mastoid antrum must begin with the preparation of the mastoid tegmen. Once the tegmen is identified, extend it forward and upward. When approaching the short process of the incus, the irrigation saline will reflect off the short process of the incus, at which point a diamond burr should be used to avoid damaging the incus. The closer you get to the head of the malleus, the greater the distance between the bony plate and the malleus-incus complex, making it safer.

3.4 How to Enlarge the Entrance of the External Auditory Canal?

When making an incision behind the ear, insert the dissector from the ear canal and extend it backward along the ear incision. Mark the upper edge of the external auditory canal, and use a small round knife to cut the skin flap along the dissector. The size of the external auditory canal opening should be such that an adult's index finger can fit through it. Suture the cut skin flap to the mastoid periosteal flap with 3-0 absorbable sutures, thus widening the external auditory canal opening.

During an endaural incision, try to reduce the height of the facial nerve ridge as much as possible, and excise the soft tissue (along with part of the cartilage) below the external auditory canal opening, and thin the skin flap of the external auditory canal to enlarge the entrance of the external auditory canal.

When packing, be sure that there are no gelatin sponges or iodoform gauze strips under the flap. Carefully clean with a suction device and probe with a dissector to ensure it is bone surface before feeling assured.

3.5 Management of Intraoperative Bleeding

Bleeding within the mastoid can be managed without irrigation by using a small diamond burr to pinpoint the bleeding site (note, this method should not be used when in close proximity to the facial nerve to avoid thermal injury to the nerve). High-temperature cauterization can be used for hemostasis. For bleeding from the tegmen bone or dura mater, bipolar coagulation can be used for hemostasis. In this case, the energy of the coagulation should be adjusted to less than half of the normal setting to prevent cerebrospinal fluid leakage. For bleeding from the sigmoid sinus, coagulation is not recommended; instead, absorbable hemostatic gauze should be used to apply pressure for hemostasis. For bleeding from the venous sinuses within the mastoid, bone wax can be used to achieve hemostasis. During cochlear implantation, the mastoid bone surface (without dura mater exposure) can be cauterized using an electric knife for hemostasis. If the dura mater is exposed, using an electric knife for hemostasis is strictly prohibited as it can easily cause meningeal damage and cerebrospinal fluid leakage.

3.6 Complications of Surgery

The most dangerous intraoperative risks that could be fatal are anesthesia accidents, massive bleeding, and brainstem injury.

The most dangerous and potentially fatal complications after surgery include infection (especially inflammatory storms), cerebrospinal fluid leakage, and various intracranial complications.

The symptoms of sigmoid sinus thrombosis can include nonspecific headaches, meningitis, and dizziness, which can be indicative. To expose the sigmoid sinus, examine its blood flow, and sometimes incise the sigmoid sinus to remove the thrombus and drain the epidural abscess. Intravenous antibiotics and heparin should be used.

3.7 Some Surgical Techniques

In some cases, the tensor tympani muscle contracts severely, causing the malleus handle to adhere closely to the promontory. It may be necessary to sever the tensor tympani tendon, which might require the removal of the incus first to expose the tensor tympani tendon.

3.7.1 How to preserve the chorda tympani nerve?

First, use an ossicle cutter to remove the head of the malleus, and then use a hook knife to cut the tendon of the tensor tympani muscle. Next, use the hook knife to separate the chorda tympani nerve from the malleus. Push the handle of the malleus forward and remove it. If the lesion near the chorda tympani nerve is difficult to remove, repeated traction may cause facial paralysis, so it is best to use a middle ear scissor to sharply cut it.

3.7.2 How to remove the upper structure of the stapes without causing a footplate fracture?

Scissor-like instruments cannot be used in this situation, as the shear force can easily lead to a fracture of the stapes footplate. A solid foundation in temporal bone anatomy training is required. I personally used six fresh temporal bone specimens before finding the appropriate force to transect the two crura of the stapes.

3.7.3 How to identify the facial nerve in the absence of obvious anatomical landmarks and without a facial nerve monitor?

This is especially challenging during revision surgery when the incus is absent and the malleus may also be difficult to locate. In such cases, the first step is to identify the sigmoid sinus and delineate the posterior boundary of the surgical field. Next, locate the tegmen (including the mastoid tegmen and the tegmen tympani) above. Generally, remnants of the tensor tympani tendon can be found in the anteroinferior area. The facial nerve lies just posterior and lateral to this tendon. Locate the promontory, and the round window can usually be found. The oval window is situated just posterosuperior to the round window. The distance from the tensor tympani tendon to the oval window is approximately equal to the distance from the oval window to the geniculate ganglion, which helps in roughly locating the facial nerve. Then, proceed from top to bottom, clearing the bone surface longitudinally in the direction of the facial nerve. Avoid operating perpendicular to the direction of the facial nerve, as this increases the risk of nerve damage. Blood vessels (striae) are often present on the surface of the facial nerve. The horizontal semicircular canal is not a very reliable landmark, especially during revision surgery.

3.7.4 How to quickly dry the ear?

First, ensure thorough removal of the lesion and smooth drainage. Open the surgical cavity, and try to reduce the height of the facial nerve ridge. The size of the external auditory canal opening should match the size of the surgical cavity. If the mastoid is well-pneumatized or even overpneumatized, materials such as cartilage, bone powder, and skin flaps should be used to narrow the surgical cavity.

After mastoidectomy, it is impossible for blood vessels to regenerate on the bone surface. Some soft tissues such as fascia, perichondrium, or thin layers of skin grafts are needed to accelerate the rate of epithelialization. Efforts should be made to minimize the exposure of the bone surface.

Try to avoid direct contact of iodoform gauze with soft tissue surfaces, as it can stimulate granulation growth. Gelatin sponge has ototoxicity; otic absorbable cotton is more effective than gelatin sponge for ear use. Covering the surgical cavity with it can reduce the time for the ear to dry. If conditions permit, medical silicone sheets can also be used.

Finally, fill the surgical cavity with iodoform gauze. Apply moderate pressure, not too tight, to avoid excessive compression that may cause dizziness, tinnitus, or even facial paralysis (when the facial nerve is exposed).

3.7.5 What Factors Affect Postoperative Hearing?

There are many factors that affect the hearing outcome after tympanoplasty, including the postoperative state of the middle ear (acoustic properties of the reconstructed tympanic membrane), the condition of the middle ear mucosa (presence of granulation tissue or secretions), surgical technique, external auditory canal resonance, tympanic cavity volume, scar formation, (inflammation-induced) annular ligament sclerosis, the surgeon's experience, individual patient differences, comorbidities (such as diabetes, cleft palate, etc.), postoperative follow-up duration, changes in cochlear function (bone conduction hearing threshold), and the healing and sound transmission characteristics of the artificial ossicles (shape, material, etc.). Current research in middle ear mechanics has been very helpful in guiding clinical practice. There are clear data on the weight of the ossicles and the angle of implantation. The resonance effect of the concha increases sound in the 4–5 kHz range by 10 dB. The geometric parameters of the external auditory canal (radius, length, volume) determine the resonance frequency. According to physical principles, a tube closed at one end can resonate with sound waves whose wavelength is four times its length. The external auditory canal is approximately 2.5 cm long, with a resonance frequency of about 2–3 kHz. After mastoidectomy, the resonance frequency changes. The sound pressure enhancement effect of the auricle is related to its shape and the angle at which sound enters, which is important for sound localization. Recent studies have found that the resonance frequency of the external auditory canal is 2800–3100 Hz, and sound pressure in the 2–4 kHz frequency range is enhanced by approximately 10 dB.

Changes in the shape of the external auditory canal after surgery can also affect its resonance frequency. After mastoidectomy, the removal of the posterior wall of the external auditory canal results in an increased volume and a lowered resonance frequency. Studies have found that the larger the entrance of the external auditory canal, the higher the resonance frequency; conversely, the larger the volume of the surgical cavity, the lower the resonance frequency. The resonance frequency of the mastoidectomy cavity decreases from 2942 Hz in normal individuals to 1939 Hz, primarily due to an increase in volume from 0.9 to 2.3 ml. The width of the entrance of the external auditory canal and the characteristics of the walls covering the surgical cavity (whether angled or smooth) have minimal impact. Due to the enlargement of the surgical cavity, the sound pressure enhancement in the 3–4 kHz range of the external auditory canal is reduced by approximately 10 dB. The fundamental frequency range of 2800–3200 Hz is critically important to the entire speech spectrum.

The reduction in the volume of the posttympanic cavity after radical surgery is another reason for changes in acoustic characteristics. The normal volume of the middle ear mastoid is approximately 6 cm^3, while the volume of the posttympanic cavity after radical surgery decreases to about 1 cm^3. The volume of a flattened tympanic cavity decreases even more (0.5 cm^3). According to experiments and calculations, this can result in a conductive hearing loss of 10 dB or even greater in the low-frequency region.

Current research has found that the placement of artificial ossicles during surgery is one of the main factors affecting postoperative hearing outcomes. If the stapes are intact, the postoperative hearing outcome with PORP placement is better than with TORP placement after the stapes superstructure is absent. This is because the stability of PORP is superior to that of TORP. If the selected ossicle is too short, scar contraction after surgery can affect hearing conduction. If it is too long, it may be expelled easily, and excessive pressure on the stapes annular ligament can also impact hearing outcomes. The optimal angle between the TORP and the tympanic membrane is not 90° but 45°. Titanium ossicles with a slightly pointed top can better integrate with cartilage, increasing stability. If the TORP is cylindrical, a small cartilage piece can be added to the footplate where it contacts the stapes footplate. Using a small suction tube to make a hole in the cartilage and fitting it onto the ossicle can increase stability.

The acoustic transmission characteristics of thin and thick cartilage plates: Thin plates have good sound transmission capabilities but lack stability. Thick plates reflect sound waves but are sufficiently stable.

The amplitude-frequency curve of the temporalis fascia and perichondrium shows characteristics of a relatively thin and soft membrane, with its resonance peak located at low frequencies. The curve of a normal tympanic membrane is relatively smooth and has good transmission capability over a wide frequency range. The frequency curve of cartilage with a thickness of less than 500 μm is very similar to that of a normal tympanic membrane, with no significant amplitude drop in the 500–1500 Hz range. Thicker cartilage shows varying degrees of amplitude reduction. The auricular cartilage layer, which is about 1 mm thick, exhibits approximately 25–30 dB hearing loss at 1 kHz.

To ensure good sound transmission in a well-ventilated middle ear cavity, the cartilage slice should be thinned as much as possible. A cartilage slice with a thickness of 500 μm will not reduce the tensile strength of the eardrum in cases of ventilation obstruction. This thickness can maximize acoustic sensitivity and stability.

Increased stiffness (adhesion, hardening) affects low-frequency hearing, while increased weight affects high-frequency hearing.

Studies have found that the frequency transition of sound pressure levels within the cochlea is relatively smooth. The movement of the malleus rotational axis, which is frequency-dependent, may smooth out the frequencies received by the tympanic membrane before transmitting them to the inner ear. The key to this smooth frequency processing is that the tympanic membrane must be fully attached to the handle of the malleus, not just at the umbo. To preserve this acoustic characteristic, surgeons should pay attention to this coupling area and avoid unnecessary loosening of it.

3.8 The Principles of Managing Related Lesions

3.8.1 Cholesterol Granuloma of the Middle Ear

It is mainly caused by dysfunction of the middle ear (mastoid) ventilation system. Temporal bone cholesterol granuloma is a yellow-brown, mucous-like lesion first described by Manasse in 1894. The most common site is the petrous apex, which is also the most common primary site. MRI can accurately diagnose it. The characteristic is high signal intensity on both T1- and T2-weighted images, with no enhancement after the application of Gd-DTPA. If the lesion shows high signal intensity only on T1-weighted images, it may indicate the presence of cholesterol crystals, protein components, and hemorrhage. MRI can distinguish cholesterol granuloma coexisting with cholesteatoma, as cholesteatoma shows high signal intensity only on T2-weighted images.

The middle ear ventilation system includes the Eustachian tube, the area around the incus (which determines the ventilation of the mastoid), and three valve structures in the epitympanic recess. Thin-slice CT scans and otoscopic examinations are very helpful in identifying the locations of ventilation obstructions.

(1) How to determine the function of the Eustachian tube: The middle ear ventilation system is a complex system, and the Eustachian tube is just one, albeit an important, component of it. Wullstein proposed long ago that the area near the incus is the second valve of the middle ear. This area determines the ventilation and drainage of the mastoid antrum and most of the mastoid cells. The anterior and posterior isthmus of the epitympanum determines the drainage of the epitympanum. Currently, there is no particularly accurate test for Eustachian tube function. Tympanometry, tympanic pressure graphs, instillation of medication through a perforated tympanic membrane, and the Valsalva maneuver are all indirect methods of examination. Wullstein even stated that the best method to examine the Eustachian tube is tympanoplasty. Professor Helms found that in over 90% of cases of otitis media and cholesteatoma during surgery, the Eustachian tube function was basically normal. From this, it can be inferred that chronic suppurative otitis media and cholesteatoma are conditions where there was a period of Eustachian tube dysfunction during childhood (the most common cause being adenoid hypertrophy), after which the Eustachian tube function recovered, but the middle ear pathology had become an irreversible condition. Otoscopy combined with CT scanning can roughly determine the location of the middle ear drainage obstruction (see the otoscopy section). If the tympanic membrane is intact and CT scans show aeration behind the tympanic membrane, it suggests that the Eustachian tube function is still adequate. The following conditions all suggest possible Eustachian tube dysfunction: cleft palate, nasopharyngeal carcinoma and postradiotherapy, hemifacial developmental anomalies, allergic rhinitis, Samter's triad, obesity, smoking, pregnancy, maxillofacial trauma and fractures, cystic fibrosis, Kartagener syndrome, and gastroesophageal reflux.

(2) How to determine the ventilation of the mastoid (second valve) when the tympanic membrane is intact: if a CT scan shows air behind the tympanic membrane but shadows in the mastoid, it suggests that the Eustachian tube function is still adequate, mainly indicating

poor drainage around the incus. If the mastoid is small, an incision inside the ear can be made to directly open the mastoid, preserving part of the bony bridge and the incus. A small piece of tragal cartilage can be used to close the mastoid antrum, allowing the mastoid to drain directly into the external auditory canal. If the mastoid is well pneumatized, or even hyperpneumatized, a postauricular incision should be made to clear as many mastoid air cells and lesions as possible. The facial recess should be opened, the incus and head of the malleus removed, and the mastoid antrum and epitympanic recess thoroughly opened. A partial ossicular replacement prosthesis (PORP) can be used to reconstruct the ossicular chain. If the external auditory canal is wide, the surgical method for otosclerosis can be referenced: remove part of the posterior inferior wall of the external auditory canal from the canal side to expose the incudostapedial joint and then remove the incus. If the canal is narrow, the mastoid and facial recess should be opened first, and then the incus should be removed.

(3) How to determine the ventilation condition of the epitympanum: If otoscopic examination reveals retraction of the pars flaccida, excessive inward retraction of the malleus handle, and close contact with the promontory, it indicates ventilation obstruction of the epitympanum. The best treatment approach is to sever the tensor tympani muscle (which often has a negative effect on epitympanic drainage) and remove the head of the malleus (in many cases, the incus needs to be removed first). If hearing preservation is a concern and the incus is not removed, the recurrence rate is high. Treating sclerosis of the tensor tympani muscle is not difficult; it can be severed with a hook knife without affecting the vibration of the tympanic membrane. Severing the tensor tympani muscle often also releases the contact between the malleus handle and the promontory.

It should be noted that Eustachian tube balloon dilation and tympanostomy tube placement both address middle ear ventilation issues but do not improve ventilation of the mastoid and epitympanic recess. Studies by Post and Bothwell indicate that biofilms within tympanostomy tubes often cause persistent and difficult-to-treat infections.

3.8.2 Adhesive Otitis Media

Some authors include atelectasis of the middle ear and adhesive otitis media in the staging system of tympanic membrane retraction, representing two progressive stages of the disappearance of the fibrous layer of the tympanic membrane: Stage I, tympanic membrane retraction; Stage II, tympanic membrane retraction with contact to the incus; Stage III, atelectasis of the middle ear; and Stage IV, adhesive otitis media [1]. Contact between the ossicles and the retracted tympanic membrane can lead to bone erosion.

Another important factor leading to middle ear atelectasis and chronic otitis media is the degree of mastoid pneumatization. The mastoid is an air-containing cavity connected to the middle ear, which often remains in a state of negative pressure during chronic otitis media. Similar to the middle ear, the mastoid acts as a pressure buffer, capable of resisting changes in middle ear pressure (according to Boyle's law). Studies by Sade and others on this closed system of the mastoid have confirmed that the smaller the mastoid air cells, the weaker its pressure buffering capacity, thereby increasing the tympanic membrane's sensitivity to the increased negative pressure in the middle ear [2].

A 5-year follow-up study found that infants treated with tympanostomy tubes for recurrent acute otitis media or chronic otitis media with effusion required multiple ventilation tubes and repeated tympanostomy tube placements. In infants with retracted tympanic membranes, this ultimately led to poor mastoid development and a corresponding reduction in the size of the air cell system [3].

In addition to Eustachian tube dysfunction, another significant cause of adhesive otitis media is tympanic membrane damage, which leads to the loss of its inherent reticular structure and elasticity, resulting in aging and laxity. This decreases its tensile strength, making it unable to resist negative pressure and causing retraction [4–6]. This reason is also a crucial factor contributing to the suboptimal efficacy of tympanoplasty.

It has been found that the complex microstructure of the eardrum, especially the central part, cannot be fully repaired after damage. Histological studies have shown that even in spontaneously healed eardrums, the arrangement of the fibrous structure does not return to normal. The lack of normal lamina propria structure and elasticity results in the loss of acoustic transmission characteristics and stability during pressure fluctuations. This suggests that invasive treatments of the eardrum, such as repeated incisions and tube placements, should be minimized to reduce damage to the eardrum's pressure receptors.

The characteristics of tympanic membrane reconstruction depend on the properties of the graft (size, quality, hardness) as well as the surgical technique (position of the graft, connection of the graft to the ossicular chain and the handle of the malleus, etc.). The hardness of different materials is compared under the same layer thickness. Temporalis fascia and perichondrium are significantly softer than the tympanic membrane. If the perforation area is large, the ability of these materials to resist static pressure changes and their stability must be considered, as they may lack sufficient stability. Retraction may occur in cases of Eustachian tube dysfunction. Cartilage is definitely thicker than the tympanic membrane; thus it is harder. Its compressive strength is related to its thickness. Cartilage with a layer thickness of 500–600 μm has a vibration curve similar to that of a normal tympanic membrane within the range of atmospheric pressure changes, meaning its hardness is comparable. Thinner cartilage of 420 μm shows a steeper curve change than the tympanic membrane, indicating it is less hard. When middle ear ventilation is normal or partially functional, thinner cartilage should be used to achieve sufficient stability. In cases of long-term Eustachian tube dysfunction with negative pressure in the middle ear, a 500 μm cartilage plate (the thickness of tragal cartilage is about 500 μm) should be used for more stable reconstruction.

To restore sufficient tension to the eardrum, it is necessary to excise the eardrum that has adhered to the tympanic cavity [7, 8]. The eardrum can be reconstructed using materials with high tensile strength, such as cartilage. Although cartilage is relatively thick and may reduce the volume of the tympanic cavity, research by Merchant et al. has shown that the total volume of the mastoid cavity is approximately 6 cm^3, and as long as the volume of the tympanic cavity is not less than 0.5 cm^3, it will not significantly affect hearing [9]. Long-term follow-up has found that, even after 10 years, cartilage implanted in the middle ear undergoes varying degrees of softening, but approximately 50% of the cartilage cells are still retained. Additionally, removing the perichondrium on the side facing the tympanic cavity helps reduce the occurrence of adhesions [10].

3.8.3 Tympanosclerosis

Tympanosclerosis is caused by recurrent otitis media, chronic otitis media, or the presence of tympanostomy tubes. Jaisingghani found that out of 150 temporal bones taken from patients with chronic otitis media, 53 (35%) exhibited tympanosclerosis. The German Society of Otorhinolaryngology, Head and Neck Surgery defines tympanosclerosis as ① a history of chronic suppurative otitis media, and ② the presence of sclerotic plaques around the ossicular chain that affect hearing, which are necessary for the diagnosis of tympanosclerosis. Simple calcification of the tympanic membrane, or calcification on the surface of the promontory or within the mastoid, as long as it is not near the ossicular chain and does not affect hearing, cannot be termed tympanosclerosis. Studies have found that scar tissue in adhesive otitis media and sclerotic plaques in tympanosclerosis contain bacteria. Therefore, it is important to avoid opening the inner ear during surgery for these conditions. The basic principles are the following:

(1) At the end of the surgery, do not use a drill or irrigation, and clean the stapes area. If inner ear exposure occurs, immediately soak the surgical cavity with steroids, stop using the drill and irrigation, and conclude the surgery as soon as possible.
(2) Handle granulation tissue and calcified plaques in the stapes area according to the surgeon's ability. The goal is not perfection but safety [11, 12].

Smyth suggested that for patients with tympanosclerosis, closing the tympanic membrane perforation surgically is sufficient, and postoperative hearing can be improved with the use of hearing aids. Marquet also believed that the stapes surgery techniques for otosclerosis should not be directly applied to middle ear surgery for otitis media, as the rate of surgery-induced deafness is higher than 4%. Gormley demonstrated that stapedectomy can lead to total deafness, with long-term follow-up showing that only 7% of patients had an air-bone gap within 21 dB, which was attributed to recurrence of the disease. If postoperative hearing improvement is unsatisfactory, patients may use hearing aids or undergo bone bridge surgery.

3.8.4 Intraoperative Complications and Reoperation

(1) Indications for reoperation are ① severe complications from the first surgery, such as facial paralysis, cerebrospinal fluid leak, sigmoid sinus rupture and bleeding, etc., ② persistent ear discharge after surgery, and ③ desire for further hearing improvement.
(2) Stapes dislocation: immediately administer 1000 mg of hydrocortisone intravenously. For partial dislocation, stop the surgery immediately and reoperate after 6 months. For complete dislocation, repair with fascia or cartilage and reoperate after 6 months.
(3) Black blood in the surgical field: make a quick judgment, often indicating venous blood, suggesting sigmoid sinus or other venous vessel injury. Management: quickly apply finger pressure, if time allows, use a piece of muscle for compression. Then use fascia + fibrinogen gel. Fully suction and expose the vessel, and then apply pressure for more than 6 min.
(4) Facial nerve injury: if it is only a thermal burn, remove the damaged bone, expose the facial nerve, and if necessary, incise the facial nerve sheath.
(5) Labyrinthine fistula: immediately administer 1000 mg of hydrocortisone intravenously.
(6) Meningeal exposure: if it is only meningeal exposure, no treatment is needed. If the exposure area is large, it can be covered with temporal muscle fascia or cartilage membrane. If the open area is >5 mm, use cartilage for repair. Immediately administer 1000 mg of hydrocortisone intravenously.
(7) How an otologist handles otogenic brain abscess intraoperatively: About half of temporal lobe abscesses are related to middle ear inflammation, while almost all cerebellar abscesses are otogenic. It is very important to accurately locate the puncture point, generally near the granulation close to the dura mater. Cerebellar abscesses are often punctured at the granulation below the sigmoid sinus. The puncture needle should neither be too thin nor too thick. If too thin, the pus will not easily flow out; if too thick, rapid outflow of pus may cause brain herniation. Generally, a 5 ml syringe is used for puncture and drainage.
(8) If brain tissue herniates into the mastoid cavity during surgery, do not attempt to reposition it, as this may cause increased intracranial pressure. Instead, excise the protruding brain tissue to prevent cerebrospinal fluid leakage, reinforce the bone defect with cartilage, and prevent reherniation.
(9) Cerebrospinal fluid otorrhea is a very dangerous condition that requires careful and prompt management. The main causes are congenital malformations, most commonly absence of the internal auditory canal floor, where cerebrospinal fluid repeatedly impacts the stapes area, eventually penetrating into the middle ear. In this case, a large piece of

temporal muscle should be used to pack the vestibule. This is also the approach during a cerebrospinal fluid gush in cochlear implantation surgery. A rare cochlear modiolus defect presents a more complex situation, often exposing the facial nerve; the packing material required is substantial. If packed too lightly, it will not hold; if packed too tightly, it may cause facial paralysis. In such cases, intraoperative facial nerve monitoring is recommended. The packing material may contact the facial nerve (possibly causing transient mild facial paralysis postoperatively) but should not exert excessive pressure. Rarely, children with cranial bone developmental disorders present the most dangerous scenario, where the entire temporal bone becomes fragile due to prolonged cerebrospinal fluid exposure, easily breaking off in large pieces. Multiple surgeries often fail to control cerebrospinal fluid leakage. In such cases, large pieces of fat and muscle must be used to seal the middle ear cavity. Even if facial paralysis may occur, it is secondary to life preservation. Once cerebrospinal fluid leakage is fully controlled, facial paralysis can be addressed later.

References

1. Sade J, Berco E. Atelectasis and secretory otitis media. Ann Otol Rhino Laryngol. 1976;85:66–72; Tos M, Poulsen G. Attic retractions following secretory otitis. Acta Otolaryngol. 1980;89:479–86.
2. Sade J. The buffering effect of middle ear negative pressure by retraction of the pars tensa. Am J Otolaryngol. 2000;21:20–3.
3. Valtonen HJ, Dietz A, Qvarnberg YH, et al. Development of mastoid air cell system in children treated with ventilation tubes for early-onset otitis media: a prospective radiographic 5-year follow-up study. Laryngoscope. 2005;115:268–73.
4. Huang D, Yang W, Jiang S, et al. The clinical observations on 110 cases of adhesive otitis media. Chin J Otolaryngol Head Neck Surg. 1996;31(2):82–5. (Chinese)
5. Huang D. Adhesive otitis media. Chin J Otolaryngol Head Neck Surg. 1996;31(4):251–3. (Chinese)
6. Hildmann H. Sonderformen der chronischen Otitis media. In: Helms J, editor. Oto-Rhino-Laryngologie in Klinik und Praxis. Band 1 Ohr. Stuttgart/New York: Georg Thieme Verlag; 1994. p. 620–1.
7. Yu L, Han C, Yu H, et al. Auricular cartilage palisade technique for repairing tympanic membrane perforation. Chin J Otolaryngol Head Neck Surg. 2001;36(3):166–8. (Chinese)
8. Milewski C. Ergebnisse der Tympanoplastik nach Verwendung von Knorpel-Perichondriumtransplantaten zum Trommelfellersatz unter ungünstigen Bedingungen. Laryngorhinootologie. 1991;70:402–4.
9. Merchant SN, McKenna MJ, Rosowski JJ. Current status and future challenges of tympanoplasty. Eur Arch Otorhiolaryngol. 1998;255:221–8.
10. Kerr AG, Byrne JE, Smyth GD. Cartilage homografts in the middle ear: a long-term histological study. J Laryngol Otol. 1973;87:1193–9.
11. Wullstein HL, Wullstein S. Tympanoplastik. Stuttgart/New York: Georg Thieme Verlag; 1986.
12. Yu L, et al. Operative therapy of the adhesive otitis media. Chin J Otolaryngol Head Neck Surg. 2004;39(1):40–3. (Chinese)

4 Surgical Principles of Cholesteatoma

Lin Han, Yuting Tao, and Lisheng Yu

4.1 Introduction

The surgical principles of cholesteatoma vary among different schools. Below, we mainly introduce the perspectives of the German school (D. Plester; J. Helms; H. Hildmann; H. Sudhoff; K. Jahnke) and some of our own observations [1, 2]. Plester described the surgical approaches for cholesteatoma in 1979 in detail and conducted a long-term follow-up research, refining the indications for canal-wall-down mastoidectomy and canal-wall-up mastoidectomy [3, 4]. Different pathogenic process and manifestations of cholesteatoma lead to varied prognosis and different choices of treatment.

4.2 Definition

The term cholesteatoma was initially coined by Johannes Muller in 1838. The matrix of cholesteatoma comprises of squamous epithelium surrounded by inflammatory fibrous tissue. Contrary to its name, cholesteatoma does not contain fat or cholesterol. It arises when epithelial tissue penetrates and impaired the middle ear and surrounded structures, resulting in adhesions, retraction, and sacculations. Da Costa (1992) and Sade (1976) observed that roughly 10% of chronic middle ear infections are combined with cholesteatoma.

Cholesteatoma was mainly classified into congenital cholesteatoma and acquired cholesteatoma due to pathogenesis.

4.3 Classifications

4.3.1 Pathogenetic Classifications

4.3.1.1 Congenital Cholesteatoma

Congenital cholesteatoma derived from epithelial remnant which has existed since embryonic development. Previously, the diagnostic criteria for congenital cholesteatoma included cholesteatoma occurring within the middle ear cavity or other parts of the temporal bone and not associated with the tympanic membrane epithelium. Derlacki specifies that congenital cholesteatoma referred to cholesteatoma grew within an intact tympanic membrane and the patient has no history of middle ear surgery, trauma, or otitis media [5]. However, congenital cholesteatoma can be associated with recurrent otitis media. Therefore, Levenson modified the diagnostic criteria to include those who complicated with otitis media [6]. Tympanic membrane perforation, otorrhea, and the history of ear surgery (including grommet insertion) are exclusive criteria for congenital cholesteatoma.

L. Han · Y. Tao · L. Yu (✉)
Department of Otorhinolaryngology, Head and Neck Surgery, People's Hospital, Peking University, Beijing, China
e-mail: 1810301239@pku.edu.cn

L. Yu (ed.), *Progress in Postauricular Administration*, Experts' Perspectives on Medical Advances,
https://doi.org/10.1007/978-981-95-5102-6_4

The pathogenesis of congenital cholesteatoma comprises several theories, including migration of epithelial cells across an intact tympanic membrane, amniotic fluid reflux, metaplasia, and ectopic epithelial tissue during embryonic development.

Morphologically, congenital cholesteatoma presents in two forms: One type resembles sand which may occur in almost every mastoid air cells, often caused by epithelium mixing into amniotic fluid and making complete clearance challenging. Another type presents as a large mass of cholesteatoma tissue which is easier to remove with a lower recurrence rate. The CT scan of congenital cholesteatoma often showed oil painting-like shadow which cannot be explained by effusion or granulations.

4.3.1.2 Acquired Cholesteatoma

Acquired cholesteatoma generally resulted from impaired self-cleaning function of middle ear or tympanic membrane perforation. There are four classic theories concerning the pathogenesis of acquired cholesteatoma.

Epithelial migration theory. Epithelium enters the middle ear through a marginal tympanic membrane perforation.

Retraction pocket theory. Persistent malfunction of the Eustachian tube leads to retraction of the tympanic membrane, generating a pocket.

Hyperplasia theory. Excessive proliferation of basal cells results in deep epithelial invagination.

Metaplasia theory. Transformation of middle ear mucosal epithelium into cholesteatoma matrix supports this notion.

The former three theories agreed with clinical and histological findings, while the metaplasia thesis awaits confirmation or exclusion.

4.3.2 Surgical Classifications

Ernst proposed a classification of cholesteatoma procedures based on different pathogenesis and intraoperative observations. He classified cholesteatoma surgeries into surgeries of the epitympanum, mesotympanum, and complete tympanum. Tos refined this classification as below [7].

4.3.2.1 Cholesteatoma of the Pars Flaccida

This term refers to cholesteatoma that occurs in the attic, marked by retraction (the bottom of the sac is visible with otoscopy) or perforation of the pars flaccida (the bottom of the sac invisible), hence also known as attic cholesteatoma. It spreads along the sinus tympani and mastoid and eventually destructs the mesotympanum.

Chronic suppurative otitis media used to be classified as simple otitis media, bone-destructive otitis media, and cholesteatomatous otitis media. However, the retraction pocket derived from obstructed ventilation of the epitympanum (such as eustachian tube dysfunction, adenoid hypertrophy, and gastroesophageal reflux) rather than suppurative inflammation. Many people can maintain this status for years without suppurative infection or otorrhea. Thus, recently revised guidelines for the diagnosis and management of chronic otitis media identify middle ear cholesteatoma as an independent disease.

The invasiveness of cholesteatoma has been widely discussed. Many state that it depends on the degree of inflammation (including pathogenic bacteria, immune status of the patient, etc.). Without secondary inflammation, attic cholesteatoma progressed more slowly compared to sinus cholesteatoma and usually extends along the lateral aspect of the malleus into the mastoid. The destruction of the ossicular chain and hearing loss usually occur at a later stage, and complications are relatively rare. One-stage hearing reconstruction is usually feasible with a generally better prognosis.

4.3.2.2 Sinus Cholesteatoma

Sinus cholesteatoma develops from the marginal perforation or posterior superior retraction and gradually expands toward the stapes, entering the attic sinus and mesotympanum. Ventilatory obstruction often arises around the handle of the malleus. The anterior tympanic antrum and mastoid are usually intact. It is related to infection and inflammation, demonstrating considerable invasiveness and advances toward the mastoid along the incus and stapes. Destruction of the ossicular chain and hearing loss may emerge at an early stage. Patients of sinus cholesteatoma get a higher risk of complications and poor prognosis.

4.3.2.3 Tensa Cholesteatoma

Adhesions or an extensive perforation of the pars tensa can lead to tensa cholesteatoma. Lesions often extend toward the tubal orifice of eustachian tube and the attic.

4.3.2.4 Epidermosis

When the epithelium develops beneath the tympanic membrane like a flat surface, it turns into a special type of cholesteatoma known as epidermosis. TB Huy proposes that epidermosis is caused by perforation proximate to the malleus [8]. Under such circumstances, the cholesteatoma grows against the malleus and is rather easy to detach. Despite a tiny perforation, the majority of the tympanic membrane should be excised to prevent epithelial regeneration medial to the tympanic membrane.

4.3.2.5 Posttraumatic Cholesteatoma

Posttraumatic cholesteatoma arises from iatrogenic (tympanocentesis, myringotomy, tympanostomy, or grommet insertion) or traumatic tympanic perforation with epithelium invading the middle ear.

4.3.2.6 Recurrent Cholesteatoma

It is of great significance for evaluating the surgery to distinguish whether the cholesteatoma is epithelial remnant or recurrence. The latter happens when the pathogenic elements remain in the middle ear, leading to new-onset cholesteatoma.

4.3.2.7 External Auditory Canal Cholesteatoma

External auditory canal cholesteatoma usually invades the inferior external auditory canal with bony necrosis beneath it. It may be associated with mechanical irritation such as frequently cleaning ears with harsh items, leading to periostitis and bony necrosis due to chronic inflammation, active epithelial growth, and deposition of keratin debris. In this instance, the self-cleansing ability of the external auditory canal is generally impaired, requiring recurrent hospital trips for cleaning.

4.4 Epidemiology

There are few epidemiological data concerning cholesteatoma. Nager (1925) evaluated 12,000 individuals with chronic otitis media and discovered that one-third of them had cholesteatoma. Harker (1977) reported an annual incidence of 6/100,000 in Iowa, USA, and the prevalence was 0.01% [9]. Tos observed that the annual incidence was 3 cases in children and 12.6 cases in adults per 100,000 individuals in Denmark [10]. In Finland (1999), the annual incidence of cholesteatoma was 9.2 per 100,000 people, with no greater incidence reported in low-income communities, and 72.4% of cholesteatoma patients experienced recurrent otitis media [11]. Jensen et al. conducted an epidemiological investigation in Denmark from 1979 to 1983 and reported an annual incidence of 10.9 cases per 100,000 individuals [12]. The cumulative risk in men (1.1%) was significantly higher than that in women (0.7%). Those with persistent Eustachian tube dysfunction were more prone to cholesteatoma, and the incidence among patients with cleft palate was 20 times greater than that in the general population. Kim observed a comparatively high incidence rate (0.5%) in South Korea, while the incidence among the Inuit population of Great Britain's Greenland was merely 0.005% [13, 14]. However, the incidence among Inuit children in Alaska was 1.1% [15]. Similarly, the incidence among the descendants of Australian Indigenous inhabitants was 0.1%, which is much higher than usual [16].

Generally, the incidence of bilateral cholesteatoma was 10–17% [17]. Hildmann reported a bilateral incidence rate of 14%. The frequency of bilateral cholesteatoma is quite low among African Americans [18]. According to the National Center for Health Statistics study in 1978, the incidence was quite low at 4.2 cases per 100,000 individuals [19]. The epidemiological characteristics may be associated with demographics, ethnicity, and professionalism of native otologists.

4.5 Histopathology

Cholesteatoma is defined by continuous growth and increasing loss of epithelium and bone structures in the middle ear, commonly accompanied with chronic inflammation. The major mechanism of the excessive proliferation of cholesteatoma epithelium still remains elusive. Previous studies indicated that the proliferation, differentiation, and metaplasia of keratinocytes in the cholesteatoma matrix as well as the activity of fibroblasts around the matrix became abnormal during the pathogenesis of cholesteatoma. These pathological alterations are resulting from the buildup and breakdown of cellular debris in the middle ear cavity. The debris might release numerous components leading to persistent growth of the cholesteatoma. Therefore, it is necessary to eliminate epithelial debris.

It is impossible to distinguish between cholesteatoma epithelium and normal external auditory canal epithelium. Rapid proliferation is an indicator of invasive growth of cholesteatoma. The epithelium loses its invasiveness with thorough clearance of lesions, efficient drainage, and enhanced ventilation of the middle ear. Without epithelial residue, the cholesteatoma epithelium can also be used to cover the mastoid cavity.

4.6 Clinical Managements

4.6.1 Retraction Pockets

Retraction pockets can grow into cholesteatomas and invade the attic, the sinus tympani, or mesotympanum, eventually leading to tensa cholesteatomas. However, only a limited number of retraction pockets will develop into cholesteatomas. Internal (such as otitis media) or external (such as chronic otitis externa or buildup of epithelium debris) inflammation stimulates papillary growth deep into the middle ear at the base of the retraction pocket, generating the cholesteatoma. As long as the self-clearing mechanism works, the epithelium will be automatically detached, and no cholesteatoma will form. Therefore, it is vital to frequently clean the retraction pocket and verify whether the bottom of the retraction pocket can be clearly viewed.

4.6.2 Epithelium of the Opened Mastoid Cavity

The epithelium of the opened mastoid cavity does not exhibit the destructiveness of cholesteatoma epithelium because detached epithelium can be discharged when drainage is unhindered. However, the discharge might be difficult in in larger surgical cavities.

4.6.3 Auditory Ossicles

Steinbach found that approximately 50% of the ossicles removed during cholesteatoma surgery and modified for the ossicular chain reconstruction were potentially inflammatory. The inflammation results from inflammatory degradation of subepithelial bone and bone canals rather than destruction of cholesteatoma epithelium. Therefore, these ossicles lack stability [20, 21]. The use of autologous ossicles can lead to cholesteatoma recurrence. Helms et al. stated that autologous ossicular reconstruction was not appropriate for patients with chronic otitis media or cholesteatomas generally [22].

4.7 Diagnosis

4.7.1 Medical History

The medical history is usually unspecific. Otorrhea might occasionally or continuously occur, with or without rotten odor. Otalgia is rare to see. Patients with cholesteatomas can remain to have dry ears for a long time and be incidentally identified in otolaryngology clinic. If the vestibular organs, auditory organs, or facial nerve are compromised, patients can present dizziness, hearing loss (conductive or sensorineural), tinnitus, and facial paralysis. Intracranial complications without prodromal signs are scarcely observed.

4.7.2 Otoscopic Examination

A complete clearance of secretions in the ear canal is significant for microscopic inspection. Retraction pockets can be spotted in patients with attic cholesteatoma. Sinus cholesteatomas generated by marginal perforation can be easily recognized, sometimes leading to retracted tympanic membrane at the incudostapedial joint. Polyps in the posterior superior section of the tympanic membrane or attic (signal polyps) can be observed sometimes. Signal polyps usually indicates cholesteatoma even without visible cholesteatoma epithelium. An intact tympanic membrane with white appearance signals the likelihood of cholesteatoma behind it. A history of previous otologic surgery predicts residual or recurrent cholesteatoma. Always be cautious about neoplasms inferior to the tympanic membrane, because the differential diagnosis include jugulotympanic paraganglioma. The blind biopsy or surgery may cause substantial bleeding.

Congenital cholesteatomas without tympanum involvement do not present distinct signs on the tympanic membrane. Some congenital cholesteatomas infiltrating the labyrinth may only appear with nonspecific dizzy symptoms. Otitis media with effusion in children may mask cholesteatoma. The ambiguous mastoid may hide extensive cholesteatoma.

Preoperative otoscopy may complement the diagnosis occasionally. Rarely, the status of ossicular chain can be checked with otoscopy in some patients with central tympanic perforations. Endoscopic examination of the middle ear via the eustachian tube is still unsatisfying. Promoted resolution in the future may be critical for recognizing residual or recurrent cholesteatoma in postsurgery visits. Endoscopy may also be used in surgery in appropriate conditions.

4.7.3 Microbiology

The most prevalent pathogens in cholesteatoma with infections include *Pseudomonas aeruginosa*, *Staphylococcus aureus*, *Proteus species*, anaerobes, and Gram-negative *cocci*. Cholesteatoma capsules are often contaminated with a mixture of different bacteria including anaerobes. When swabbing for microbiological culture, it is of great significance to avoid mixing the specimen with the normal flora of the external auditory canal.

The therapeutic principle for cholesteatoma is surgery. Antibiotics are merely used for complications or postoperative inflammation. Otogenic brain abscesses due to cholesteatoma commonly involve anaerobic bacteria such as *Bacteroides*.

4.7.4 Fistula Symptoms

Cholesteatoma may erode the semicircular canals and 90% of the cases involves the horizontal semicircular canal. Nystagmus can be observed when performing Politzer maneuver and changing the pressure in the external auditory canal. However, these symptoms are not stable, and negative results of the fistula test do not rule out semicircular canal erosion. Among 56 cases described by Kleinsasser, only 61% of patients with surgically verified fistula exhibited positive fistula symptoms, and 10 patients had preoperative inner ear involvement. Even if the horizontal semicircular canal is entirely destroyed, fistula tests may show negative results, and patients may not present with severe hearing loss. This may be related to semicircular canal ossification which protects the inner ear. If extensive lesion exists or the posterior wall of the external auditory canal has been badly injured by previous surgery, probing the fistula area with instruments may produce fistula symptoms.

4.7.5 Audiology

Verification of pure-tone audiological results by tuning forks is important. If there is a large difference in hearing between the two sides, especially if there is severe sensorineural hearing loss on the affected side, masking may not be complete during audiometry. It is crucial to perform speech recognition testing with the unaffected side masked for assessing the exact audiological status on the affected side, and figuring out whether surgery can improve hearing. For patients with poor speech discrimination at high frequencies, surgery may not considerably ameliorate the hearing. Patient counseling should include the possibility of sound conduction via the cholesteatoma (pseudohearing) if the preoperative air-bone gap is narrow. Even if the ossicular chain is intact, surgeons may still need to remove part of it when cholesteatoma invades the ossicles. Speech audiometry can provide better evidence. Auditory brainstem response (ABR) may be applied in children or handicapped people. The otoacoustic emission test is not of great value.

4.7.6 Eustachian Tube Function Test

There are no reliable methods to assess Eustachian tube function before tympanoplasty at present. Eustachian tube dysfunction is common in patients with craniofacial abnormalities (especially in cleft palate). Dysfunction of the orofacial muscles can also induce comparable symptoms, such as Down syndrome (causing craniofacial abnormalities and orofacial muscular dysfunction that impact Eustachian tube function). Mild abnormalities of the midface can also influence nasopharyngeal ventilation and consequently produce Eustachian tube dysfunction. It has been proven that the premolar distance is related to Eustachian tube width in individuals with narrow midface, and individuals with higher hard palates have shorter nasal septa and narrower nasal cavities compared to normal humans. Koch reported that two-thirds of patients with adherent otitis media have impaired Eustachian tube function. This is also the cause of obstructed middle ear ventilation and decreased tympanic membrane flexibility and recoil.

The role of Eustachian tube dysfunction in the genesis of cholesteatomas has not been clarified. A 6-month postoperative follow-up study of 123 cholesteatoma patients indicated that 3.2% of patients showed recurrent tympanic membrane perforations. Patients with mastoiditis even had a greater recurrence risk. Recurrent perforations in this study were not produced by residual or recurrent cholesteatomas, because the latter occurred after a prolonged period postoperatively. This result indicated that Eustachian tube dysfunction is unusual in cholesteatomas and related middle ear lesions. Many famous otolaryngologists, such as Fisch and Helms, demonstrated that the proportion of Eustachian tube dysfunction proven by surgery in chronic suppurative otitis media and cholesteatomas is generally no higher than 5%. This shows that individuals with these diseases might experience Eustachian tube dysfunction at some point during childhood (such as adenoid hypertrophy). The dysfunction recovers in maturity, but middle ear lesions remain.

The latest theory is that gastric reflux is the most essential element in Eustachian tube dysfunction and otitis media with effusion. It is notable that gastroesophageal reflux is also the most important factor in adenoid hypertrophy and recurrent rhinosinusitis in children.

4.7.7 Radiology

Routine CT scans should be conducted preoperatively. CT scans can indicate the extension of the lesion, including labyrinth fistula and bony destruction. The high resolution CT can identify ossicular chain damage. Patients with anterior displacement of the sigmoid sinus often needs a transcanal technique. X-rays of Stenvers view can reflect the position of the petrous apex and sigmoid sinus and the degree of mastoid pneumatization. Canal-wall-down technique is meaningless with hypopneumatization of the mastoid air cells. However, X-rays can hardly illustrate the extent of the lesion. The MRI images of cholesteatomas lack specificity, with low signal intensity on T1-weighted images and high signal intensity on T2-weighted images. After contrast delivery, T1-weighted images can indicate the boundaries of the lesion, which is associated with granulations around the cholesteatoma. With suspicious intracranial complications or extensive lesions, the MRI can help differentiate between cholesteatomas and tumors.

4.8 Surgical Techniques

4.8.1 Anesthesia

Local anesthesia along with sedation (monitored anesthesia care, MAC) or general anesthesia is typically employed in adults.

4.8.2 Basic Principles and Techniques

The most fundamental surgical principles are the following:

(1) Complete excision of the cholesteatoma to prevent residue or recurrence.
(2) Ensuring the drainage.
(3) Preserving or reconstructing function (such as hearing function and preservation of the posterior wall of the external auditory canal). If the cholesteatoma invades the ossicular chain, sacrificing part of the ossicular chain may be essential to assure safety. In circumstances where the labyrinth fistula or cholesteatoma invades the labyrinth, compromising inner ear function may be inevitable.

4.8.3 Surgical Approach

4.8.3.1 Attic Cholesteatoma

The surgery of localized attic cholesteatomas can begin with the transcanal approach. According to Professor Helms, it is necessary to incise the mastoid following the pathology. For individuals with mastoid hypopneumatization, an approach front to back is performed. If the pneumatization is moderate, a tiny hole is created in the area of the epitympanum using a small drill bit to explore the extent of the cholesteatoma. If the sinus tympani is involved, sufficient enlargement is essential. Endoscopic inspection can be occasionally utilized to check whether cholesteatoma has been entirely excised especially in locations difficult to access with a microscope (such as the sinus tympani). This method minimizes bone removal and facilitates postoperative rebuilding. Cartilage from the tragus and attached perichondrium are used to restore the scutum. Notably, it has been confirmed that osteoclasts exist in the ossicles proximate to or wrapped in the cholesteatoma epithelium and granulations. Additionally, attic retraction pockets form due to obstructed ventilation and drainage of the epitympanum. Therefore, preserving the malleus is not suggested. To remove the malleus, the incus should be excised and the head of malleus head is removed, while the malleus handle should be preserved as much as possible. The tensor tympani muscle is often transected to elevate the tympanic membrane tightly attached to the promontory. The malleus handle should also be removed if there is cholesteatoma underneath it. The dissection should be conducted carefully to preserve the chorda tympani nerve especially with bilateral Cholesteatoma. Partial ossicular replacement titanium prosthesis (PORP) is employed to reconstruct the ossicular chain. For the initial cholesteatoma surgery, minor defects of the scutum can be repaired by tragus cartilage, and cartilage strips or thinned cartilage slices are used to reinforce the posterior tympanic membrane. The perichondrium lateral to the tympanic membrane is preserved. This approach allows stable ventilation of the epitympanum.

4.8.3.2 Sinus Cholesteatoma

The transcanal approach affords superior exposure of the sinus tympani compared to the postauricular method. The upper layers of the stapes are often involved, and the mastoid can be badly eroded. Consequently, the total ossicular replacement prosthesis (TORP) is often necessary for auditory reconstruction. However, PORP usually works better than TORP in hearing construction. If the stapedial base is deformed, such as weakening, reinforcement with cartilage membrane or temporalis muscle fascia may be required. If it is impaired, the reconstruction depends on the degree of inflammation. For cholesteatoma without severe inflammation, a thorough excision can be performed without destructing the inner ear. However, with inflammation and the inner ear structures (including the horizontal semicircular canal, the promontory and the tympanic bone) impaired, the secondary operation should be considered to prevent labyrinthitis that can lead to total deafness. After the cholesteatoma is totally excised, a small piece of cartilage with perichondrium is employed to cover the vestibular window as a new stape and the TORP is inserted.

4.8.4 Canal-Wall-Up and Canal-Wall-Down Techniques

The concept of canal-wall-up or canal-wall-down was initially established for postoperative dressing changes rather than cholesteatoma removal. Some surgeons misunderstand this notion and determine the approach before cholesteatoma removal, and this can lead to cholesteatoma residue. It is crucial to analyze the formation of cholesteatoma and evaluate whether the pathogenic factors persist when choosing the technique. Factors such as mastoid pneumatization, Eustachian tube function, age, follow-up feasibility, and contralateral ear status are critical for optimal technique selection. The location and extent of the lesion should also be considered. Additionally, the experience or preference of the surgeon greatly impact the choice in clinical practice.

Generally, the canal-wall-up technique can be employed under such circumstances: well-mastoid pneumatization, normal Eustachian tube function, children, feasible follow-ups, or limited lesions. Canal-wall-down procedures are preferably utilized with poor mastoid pneumatization (sclerotic mastoid), anterior displacement of the sigmoid sinus, tegmen mastoideum sagging, Eustachian tube malfunction, elderly patients, difficulties in follow-up, or extensive lesions. Long-term follow-up observation has demonstrated that adopting diverse approaches for different types and extents of cholesteatoma can yield better outcomes. The recurrence rate is significant for beginners and canal-wall-up surgeries, so it is crucial to maintain surgical indications conduct the surgery by highly experienced surgeons.

Hildmann characterized canal-wall-up procedures as those that conserve or reconstruct the posterior ear canal wall and obtain mastoid ventilation [1]. This guarantees the normal depth of the tympanic cavity and ordinary vibration of the ossicular chain. Removing the bony posterior canal wall and inserting it into the mastoid after mastoidectomy, or utilizing techniques similar to this with cartilage, does not constitute a canal-wall-up technique due to the lack of vented sinus tympani.

Canal-wall-up procedures are generally useful for traumatic or congenital cholesteatomas of the mesotympanum with normal middle ear ventilation. When the fracture line crosses the Eustachian tube, the canal-wall-up method cannot be employed. With comprehensive understanding of the patient (the anatomy and lesion), skilled techniques, normal Eustachian tube function, and total excision of cholesteatoma, canal-wall-up approaches can virtually retain or restore normal middle ear function. Cartilage from the tragus or auricle is routinely used to repair the posterior ear canal wall.

The absolute criteria for canal-wall-down methods include a small mastoid, inadequate mastoid pneumatization, or anterior displacement of the sigmoid sinus. With Eustachian tube dysfunction, hearing preservation is not advised. If it is not possible to completely remove the cholesteatoma in the mastoid, a canal-wall-down method is necessary. For elderly patients, the canal-wall-down procedure should be preferred whenever possible. If follow-up cannot be ensured, this technique is much safer. Under all the above circumstances, efforts should be made to narrow the surgical cavity to improve its self-cleansing capabilities. Traditional radical mastoidectomy is no longer performed. The mesotympanum should be blocked up in principle. If the posterior ear canal wall is intact or repaired, a reexploration surgery is required after 1 year postoperatively in children or 2 years in adults. Due to residual cholesteatoma growing slowly, it will be difficult to diagnose if the resurgery is performed in a short period.

The decision on surgical technique should be made preoperatively. While conducting the canal-wall-down technique, the posterior and/or superior canal wall is gradually removed along the cholesteatoma until the lesion is entirely revealed. This procedure is suitable for both poorly and normal pneumatized mastoids. The latter can recover self-cleansing capacity right after surgery with a low recurrence rate. However, in cases of excessive mastoid pneumatization, the surgery will be challenging and time-consuming, and dry ears will be difficult to accomplish.

The basic approach to achieve a small mastoid cavity capable of self-cleansing is to enlarge the external auditory canal opening sufficiently. Partial excision of the cartilage of the ear canal can be conducted, and the dorsal perichondrium can be used to cover the mastoid and restrict the surgical cavity. Certainly, the bone at the opening of external auditory canal should be removed as much as possible. After complete removal of the cholesteatoma, the facial nerve ridge is trimmed and stretched downward. The surgical cavity is flattened with a diamond bur to ensure there are no bone ridges. These techniques are enough for mastoids with poor pneumatization.

The cortical bone should be excised down to the sigmoid sinus when the mastoid is excessively pneumatized to significantly reduce the height of the operative cavity. The bone not proximate to the cholesteatoma can be kept during grinding to narrow the surgical cavity. Additionally, the mastoid tip should be cleansed until a thin and movable bony plate is preserved, which is linked to the sternocleidomastoid muscle. This method can further reduce the surgical cavity and ensure the self-cleansing ability even after canal-wall-down surgery for highly pneumatized mastoids.

To promote the epithelialization of the surgical cavity, the cholesteatoma epithelium that has been excised or detached can be put back into the surgical cavity. However, this is only applicable the cholesteatoma epithelium gets no inflammation and is put on a smooth bony surface without closed air cells beneath.

4.8.5 Packing Techniques

Before packing, the cholesteatoma must be entirely removed. If there is any possible residual, only cartilage with perichondrium should be used to cover the surgical cavity. Techniques of operative cavity reduction are generally employed for revision operations and seldom for original surgeries. Revision operation provides the chance to ensure the cholesteatoma epithelium has been fully cleansed and remove inflammatory tissue in the surgical cavity.

Common packing materials for mastoid include the Palva flap, bone powder, cartilage, and bony substitute materials (tricalcium phosphate-bioglass ceramics, BMP, etc.). The Palva myoperiosteal flap was firstly documented by Leland in the early twentieth century and was observed to get commonly scarred in revision procedures. This is not a disadvantage as scarring helps maintain its size relatively steady. Bony powder can be gathered by glass connecting tubes connected to aspirators or dissectors invented by Freer. Bone powder can be used to pack the semicircular canals and bone grooves surrounding the attic and labyrinth which are hardly visible. Small bone grooves can also be mended by cartilage with perichondrium. Bioglass ceramics, such as tricalcium phosphate bioglass ceramics, can be employed as bone substitute materials for complete or partial packing of the mastoid cavity. If this material is extensively used, its surface must be covered by cartilage with perichondrium or myoperiosteal flaps. In cases when a major mastoid cavity is created by the initial surgery, it should be narrowed during revision surgery. Instead of reducing the facial nerve ridge excessively, bioglass ceramics can be utilized to fill deep bone grooves. If the dura mater is widely exposed, artificial dura mater mixed with bioglass ceramics can also be employed.

4.8.6 Reconstruction of the Ossicular Chain

The principles of ossicular chain reconstruction in cholesteatoma surgery do not differ considerably from that of tympanoplasty. Generally, autologous ossicles cannot be modified for hearing reconstruction. The commonly used materials in Europe for prosthetic ossicles include metal and bioceramic. The choice of artificial ossicle material is explored in the chapter on artificial ossicles.

Autologous or allogeneic ossicles may stick to or even fuse with the stapes, making separation difficult in reoperation. This is worth attention in cholesteatoma surgeries. Artificial ossicles, on the other hand, are easy to separate. Cholesteatoma excision and hearing reconstruction should be done in a single-stage procedure in principle. A second surgery is only considered in specific conditions. For example, if the epithelium between the oval window and the stapes footplate cannot be reliably removed, phased surgery may be considered. During reoperation, the epithelium generates epithelial pearls which is easy to separate. Due to lack of nutrition, residual cholesteatoma of a small amount may vanish on its own. If it is difficult to attain satisfying hearing outcomes by one-stage surgery, a second surgery to improve hearing may be necessary.

Using cartilage grafts between artificial ossicles and the tympanic membrane as a routine can eliminate expulsion reaction, reduce retraction pockets, and decrease recurrence. In classic type III tympanoplasty, inserting a cartilage graft above the head of the stapes can increase the tensile strength of the tympanic membrane and improve oval window ventilation. This technique is typically employed in opened mastoid cavities. The round window is generally covered with a cartilage graft linked to perichondrium to assure the optimal sound transmission and reliable ventilation in classic type IV tympanoplasty. Additionally, the condition of the contralateral side should also be considered before operation. The reconstruction cannot be performed when there are granulations on the oval window or the footplate of the stapes.is impaired.

4.8.7 Tympanic Membrane Repair

Currently, only autologous tissue such as fascia, perichondrium, or cartilage can be used to mend the tympanic membrane.

4.8.7.1 Temporal Muscle Fascia

The fascia is easy to harvest, and there is rarely fibrous layer that contributes to scarring. Moreover, the operation is straightforward, and the fascia can adhere tightly to the lower edge of the tympanic membrane. The drawback is that temporal muscle fascia is thinner than cartilage and tends to atrophy.

4.8.7.2 Perichondrium

The perichondrium can be extracted from the tragus cartilage or auricular cartilage. Despite its toughness, its adhesion to the tympanic membrane is not as good as temporal muscle fascia; thus cautious operation is required. The problem is that the size of the perichondrium extracted from the tragus cartilage is limited, and another incision is required.

4.8.7.3 Cartilage

There are now several methods using cartilage. The side of perichondrium facing the tympanum is generally detached to minimize middle ear adhesions. The advantage of cartilage lies in the strong tensile strength to prevent retraction pockets and atrophy. It is particularly suitable for major perforations, Eustachian tube dysfunction, and adhesive otitis media. When utilizing artificial ossicles, inserting cartilage grafts can minimize the expulsion reaction of artificial ossicles. The perichondrium and cartilage island flap shows the best vibrational performance. The cartilage can be thinned as needed, and cartilage thinning devices are available now.

The palisade technique is another method that can assure adequate vibration and moderate tensile strength. The cartilage is sliced into five strips, each 1.5–2mm in width, with perichondrium on the side facing the ear canal. This material is more difficult to operate than utilizing fascia or perichondrium especially when there is severe tympanic retraction. Cartilage is thicker than other materials; hence it can decrease the volume of the tympanic cavity. Also, it is difficult to elevate the tympanomeatal flap during reoperation, and the cartilage implanted previously often needs to be removed and replaced. Epithelial invasion can occur between the cartilage palisades, so caution should be paid to the tight arrangement of the cartilage strips. Another drawback of the palisade technique is that it is not easy to observe the residual or recurrent cholesteatoma.

4.8.8 Reoperation

It is vital to perform a reoperation following a canal-wall-up surgery. Another rationale for a secondary operation is hearing promotion, although the first-time surgery should enhance hearing function as much as feasible.

The main surgical indications for reoperation include recurrent cholesteatoma, tympanic membrane perforation, needs of hearing promotion, postoperatively persistent otorrhea, and early or late complications (such as meningoencephalocele).

It is necessary to analyze the pathogenic factor and the details of the previous surgery. Special attention should be paid to Eustachian tube function. Recurrent tympanic membrane perforation and extensive adhesions may suggest Eustachian tube dysfunction, making it tough to provide ventilation of the mastoid even with reoperation. Under such circumstances, canal-wall-down procedures or mastoid occlusion may be preferred. It can be difficult to discern between residual and recurrent cholesteatoma sometimes.

4.8.9 Residual Cholesteatoma

With severe inflammation and epithelium attached to fistula of the cochlea or semicircular canals, opening the inner ear may lead to complete deafness. Therefore, it is permissible to temporarily retain the cholesteatoma epithelium and clean it during a second-stage surgery. This is the only scenario where a small amount of cholesteatoma epithelium is deliberately retained during the initial surgery.

Majorly, residual cholesteatoma is not a deliberate choice rather a consequence of limited visibility. Therefore, it is necessary to broaden the vision during the procedure to ensure visibility in every corner. For extensive cholesteatomas in well-pneumatized mastoids, extended mastoidectomy with facial recess approach is usually employed, and canal-wall-up technique (Jansen or so-called IBM surgery) has been abandoned now.

Residual cholesteatoma is often discovered during reoperation. Recurrence of facial palsy, dizziness, or hearing loss after surgery may indicate residual cholesteatoma. Radiological examinations aid in early detection of cholesteatoma. Small- or flat-growing cholesteatomas are difficult to detect postoperatively due to anatomical changes. Exploration through a small opening in the mastoid or sinus tympani can also be performed.

There are no specific surgical principles for managing residual cholesteatoma. However, in cases where previous surgery involved cholesteatoma, all parts of the middle ear must be inspected during reoperation. Common sites for residual cholesteatoma include the attic (often in the anterior portion), and sometimes epithelial pearls can be observed in the mesotympanum. Residual cholesteatoma in the inferior epitympanic recess and mastoid is less common but challenging to tackle with as they may invade the superior, posterior, and inferior labyrinth. Due to their deep location and extensive nature, thorough exploration is time-consuming, and postoperative functional reconstruction is often required. Rarely, exposure of the middle or posterior cranial fossa meninges may be necessary to achieve better visualization of cholesteatoma around the labyrinth.

If the previous surgery confirmed the cholesteatoma was confined to the mesotympanum and there is suspicious residual cholesteatoma around the oval window, the oval window can be exposed through the external auditory to directly check if there is any residual cholesteatoma.

4.8.10 Recurrent Cholesteatoma

Recurrence is primarily due to Eustachian tube dysfunction, inadequate reinforcement or restoration of the superior posterior canal wall, cartilage strip lateralizing, etc. After complete excision of the epithelial sac, the decision between canal-wall-up and canal-wall-down procedures depends on Eustachian tube function. Long-term follow-up is important especially in adolescents and kids, as recurrence might occur even many years after surgery.

If recurrent cholesteatoma occurs as tensa cholesteatoma or sinus cholesteatoma, it is significant to reconstruct the tympanic membrane using cartilage and pay attention to the distance between cartilage and promontory. While utilizing palisade technique, the strips should be tightly replaced to prevent the epithelium invades the middle ear through the fissure and leads to recurrent cholesteatoma.

4.8.11 Persistent Otorrhea

Indications for reoperation include inadequate visualization of the operative cavity, residual or recurrent cholesteatoma, or continuous discharge. Recurrent perforation and secondary prolonged inflammation leading to inadequate epithelialization are the main reasons of persistent otorrhea. Moreover, obstructed drainage of the surgical cavity due to incomplete opening of impaired air cells can lead to consistent ear discharge. Before reoperation, thoroughly cleansing the surgical cavity and analyzing the underlying causes of chronic otorrhea are necessary. The reoperation needs to achieve these goals:

(1) A wide opening of external auditory canal
(2) Complete epithelialization of the tympanic membrane and external auditory canal
(3) Avoiding excessive height of the facial nerve ridge
(4) Self-cleansing capacity of the mastoid cavity
(5) No visible residual cholesteatoma

If microscopy cannot guarantee visualization, endoscopy can be utilized for further investigation. The postauricular approach is suitable for reoperation to grant visibility. Care must be made to avoid injuring the exposed sigmoid sinus. Unopened air cells should be methodically opened, the facial nerve ridge should be decreased, and the drainage from the mastoid to the external auditory canal should be kept unobstructed. The canal-wall-down technique should be adopted. If canal-wall-up or packing procedures are employed, the facial nerve ridge should not be severely trimmed. It is vital to guarantee full removal of cholesteatoma epithelium, as packing materials such as bone powder or bioceramics may be mingled with epithelium.

4.8.12 Congenital Cholesteatoma in Children

Reoperation for a second look is advised 1–2 years after the initial surgery.

4.9 Complications

Patients should be informed that cholesteatoma is a potentially fatal disease, and the primary goal of the first operation is a complete lesion excision, while functional reconstruction depends on inoperative findings. The reconstruction should usually be done in a single-stage surgery. However, a second-stage hearing reconstruction is sometimes inevitable. This should be explained to parents of children and adolescents. Besides, preoperative examinations should exclude inner ear lesions.

Good visibility is vital for the operation. The external auditory canal should be enlarged first. Removing the skin from the posterior wall of the external auditory canal allows the use of a drill. The excised skin flap can be replaced back to cover bone surfaces without impeding healing. For extensive cholesteatomas, anatomical landmarks should be identified at an early stage. The facial nerve should be located lateral to the oval window, and its route within the mastoid should be confirmed. The facial nerve ridge should be trimmed until the facial nerve is almost visible through the thinned bone, assuring speedy and safe operation.

4.9.1 Dural Exposure and Brain Herniation

Small dural exposures pose little threat, while extensive ones can lead to brain herniation. If the tegmen tympani defect exceeds 1 cm, it should be reinforced with cartilage or bone. Antibiotics should be routinely given if the dura is injured. For brain herniation, the protruding brain tissue should be removed and the defect treated with fascia or other materials before reinforcing with cartilage or bone. Replacing the herniated tissue back can aggravate the condition.

4.9.2 Labyrinthine Fistula

Not all patients with labyrinthine fistula present with positive fistula symptoms before surgery. Over 90% of labyrinthine fistulas involve the horizontal semicircular canal, and extensive cholesteatomas may involve other semicircular canals as well. Epithelium rarely penetrates the semicircular canals. Cholesteatoma can develop insidiously ventral to the superior semicircular canal or surrounding the labyrinth. Gently pushing the stapes may reveal pulsations at the exposed fistula. Grading of the fistula is important. Cholesteatoma epithelium around the fistula should be excised. The underwater technique can be utilized, which means filling the surgical cavity with saline solution and operate underwater to maintain inner ear function even when fistulas are large. After thorough excision of cholesteatoma, the fistula can be filled with bone powder and closed with perichondrium. Ossification of packed semicircular canals normally completes within 6 months. Canal-wall-down procedures are generally not recommended for patients with labyrinthine fistulas. Notably, even with semicircular canals badly injured, some patients still have hearing function.

4.9.3 Facial Nerve Exposure

The exposed facial nerve can be observed during surgery of extensive cholesteatoma with no preoperative facial palsy. Over 50% of such patients are with labyrinthine fistulas. In complex cases, the facial nerve can be identified by the position of the promontory, the oval window, and round window. Intraoperative facial nerve monitoring is not necessary.

If the facial nerve is impaired, immediate reconstruction should be performed. For partial injury, surgeons can cut off the facial nerve and take the auricular nerve for grafting. Researches concerning facial nerve combing for facial nerve spasm found that after excising part of the nerve, the function can be well restored. Thus, if the nerve is completely severed, end-to-end anastomosis is better than nerve grafting.

4.9.4 Sigmoid Sinus Thrombosis and Otogenic Sepsis

Once the sigmoid sinus is exposed, the bone above it should be thinned and the notch should be mended with perichondrium-covered cartilage. Tiny injuries of the sigmoid sinus, such as those produced by punctures, can be addressed with absorbable gelatin sponge or tiny muscle patches. Larger injuries may necessitate packing.

Sigmoid sinus thrombosis is primarily caused by surrounding inflammation. Diagnosis is accomplished by MRI with contrast imaging. MRI can reveal other intracranial lesions such as edema. Middle ear lesions should be cleansed initially. Sigmoid sinus puncture is necessary for severe infection. A small dose of heparin should be employed once thrombosis is confirmed, and only if there is concurrent infection should the jugular vein be ligated to prevent sepsis. Postoperative otogenic cerebral edema should be considered.

4.9.5 Meningitis and Brain Abscess

Otogenic meningitis develops from chronic middle ear infections migrating to the brain via deteriorated bone, arteries, nerves, or the labyrinth. Cholesteatoma, the source of otogenic meningitis or brain abscess, must be eliminated. After complete excision of cholesteatoma from the mastoid and epitympanum, the tegmen tympani should be cleansed with drill, and its defects which may cause intracranial lesions should be recognized. It is vital to figure out whether extradural abscess exists. A high dose of antibiotics that can penetrate the blood-brain barrier should be applied. If brain abscess is confirmed, neurosurgeons should participate. The treatment depends on conditions of the patient, the location, and the size and maturity of abscess. Percutaneous drainage under imaging guidance is the ideal treatment for brain abscess. Exploratory punctures are not recommended due to the possibility of infection spreading and aggravated brain damage.

4.9.6 Epidural Abscess

Epidural abscesses require a total exposure until normal dura mater is reached, followed by drainage. Under such circumstances, the posterior wall of the external auditory canal should be kept. Otherwise, the inner table of skull will be proximate to the infected mastoid.

4.9.7 Residual Hearing Ear

Cholesteatoma surgery can lead to complete deafness. Surgery on ears with residual hearing should be particularly careful. For extensive cholesteatomas, separation of the incudostapedial joint should be performed early, and operations for hearing enhancement around the stapes should be abandoned. If ossicular chain reconstruction is undertaken, a dependable approach should be adopted, such as the classic type III tympanoplasty with cartilage grafting on the artificial ossicles. Artificial ossicles should be of good stability. In principle, the surgery for residual ear should be undertaken in hospitals where middle ear surgery is routinely performed by experienced surgeons.

4.9.8 Elderly Patients with Cholesteatoma

There is no maximum age limit from anesthesia for surgery in elderly patients with cholesteatoma. The chance of complications increases dramatically among elderly patients with cognition and perceptual disorders in nursing homes. These individuals cannot notice their symptoms and poorly communicate with others, and their hearing loss is mostly attributed to age-related hearing loss rather than cholesteatoma or otitis media. Regular medical examinations are not common for these seniors and the definitive diagnosis is usually delayed. For elderly patients, canal-wall-down surgery should be the first choice, as the majority of them have poor mastoid pneumatization. The recurrence rate after surgery in patients over 60 years of age is quite low. Hearing aids can be used to promote hearing in these patients.

4.9.9 Pediatric Cholesteatoma

Many experts state that cholesteatoma of children is more invasive than that of adults. Sheehy et al. evaluated 181 cases of pediatric cholesteatoma, of which 8 cases had fistula and 1 case got facial paralysis. No intracranial complications were found. On the contrary, the proportion of complications in adults with cholesteatoma was actually higher. Studies on growth factors such as EGF, TGF-α, and FGF-2 within the inflammatory capsule of cholesteatoma have revealed their association with the degree of inflammation but not with age. Mastoid pneumatization may be related to genetics and mastoid sclerosis caused by mastoiditis. Mastoids of children frequently contain more air cells, and cholesteatoma epithelium can invade them. This is an anatomical basis for the increased proportion of invasive cholesteatoma in children. In conclusion, complications such as ossicular chain impairment do not differ between adults and children, and the invasiveness depends on mastoid pneumatization, the duration, and inflammation of the cholesteatoma capsule. Additionally, better mastoid pneumatization in children leads to higher proportion of residual cholesteatoma. Persistent Eustachian tube dysfunction may also contribute to residue. Pediatric cholesteatoma is difficult to diagnose preoperatively, and if they do not heal immediately after surgery, dressing changing for children can be a tough work especially for younger ones. Generally, canal-wall-up surgery should be used for all pediatric patients, with a second look 1–2 years later. This can help kids maintain a normal life and considerably lessen the difficulty of dressing changing. Actually, even with canal-wall-down surgery, the recurrence rate of mesotympanum cholesteatoma is high due to its narrow scope, often necessitating a second surgery. Due to bone regeneration in children, canal-wall-down surgery promotes self-cleaning of the surgical cavity but narrows the cavity which eventually diminishes visibility.

Recurrent cholesteatoma grows toward the sinus tympani, and a second canal-wall-down surgery is recommended. If epithelium has been completely removed, the Palva flap can be utilized to narrow the operative cavity.

Primary congenital cholesteatoma is clearly a distinct form. According to Michael's research, the most typical location of congenital cholesteatoma in children is the anterior superior tympanum, and the initial symptom is generally tympanic effusion. Physical examination shows a faint white appearance below the handle of the malleus. If it is observed at an early stage, mastoidectomy is often not required. Sometimes cholesteatoma arises from the front of cochleariform process, and the handle of the malleus should be removed and ossicular chain reconstruction is required. Canal-wall-up surgery is indicated for congenital cholesteatoma, and a second look is often inevitable. Only in cases of persistent Eustachian tube dysfunction is canal-wall-down surgery recommended.

Pediatric and adolescent cholesteatoma patients should be followed up by a specialist, preferably the surgeon himself/herself, to detect cholesteatoma recurrence as early as possible. The major goal of secondary surgery is to discover whether there is any residual or recurrent cholesteatoma and to restore hearing function. The significance of follow-up examinations should be emphasized preoperatively in patients who cannot be followed up.

References

1. Hildmann H, Sudhoff H, Jahnke K. Grundzuege einer differenzierten Cholesteatom-Chirurgie. Laryngo-Rhino-Otologie. 2000;79(Supplement 2):73–94.
2. Hildmann H, Sudhoff H. Middle ear surgery. Berlin/Heidelberg/New York: Springer; 2006.
3. Plester D. Chirurgie des Cholesteatom. Arch Oto Rhino Laryngol. 1979;223:380–90.
4. Jahke K, Khatib M, Rau U. Langzeitergebnisse nach Cholesteatomchirurgie. Lar Rhinol Otol. 1985;64:238–42.
5. Derlacki E, Clemis JD. Congenital cholesteatoma of the middle ear and mastoid. Ann Otol Rhinol Laryngol. 1965;74:706–27.
6. Levenson MJ, Parisier SC, Chute P, et al. A review of twenty congenital cholesteatoma of the middle ear in children. Otolaryngol Head Neck Surg. 1986;94:560–7.
7. Tos M. Manual of middle ear surgery. Vol 1. Approaches, myringoplasty, ossiculoplasty and tympanoplasty. Georg Thieme Verlag; 1995. p. 102–110.
8. Tran Ban Huy P, Asienberg N. Cholesteatoma and cholesteatomas. In: Ars B, editor. Pathogenesis in cholesteatoma. Elsevier Science; 1999. p. 19–35.
9. Harker LA. Cholesteatoma: an incidence study. In: McCabe B, Sade J, Abramson M, editors. Cholesteatom: first international conference. Birmingham: Aesculapius Publishing company; 1977. p. 308–12.
10. Tos M. Incidence, etiology and pathogenesis of cholesteatoma in children. Ann Otol Rhinol Laryngol. 1988;40:110–7.
11. Kemppainen HO, Puhakka HJ, Laippala PJ, et al. Epidemiology and etiology of middle ear cholesteatoma. Acta Otolrhinollaryngol (Stockh). 1999;119:568–72.
12. Jensen HF, Vase P, Green A, et al. Cholesteatoma, an epidemiological study. In: Sanna M, editor. Proceedings of the Fifth International Conference on cholesteatoma and mastoid surgery. Roma: CIC Edizioni Internationali; 1997. p. 184–7.
13. Kim CS, Jung HW, Won HA, et al. A prevalence study of otitis media and related disease in Korea, 1991. In: Nakano Y, editor. Proceedings of the Fourth International Conference on cholesteatoma and mastoid surgery, Niigata, Japan. Amsterdam: Kugel & Gehdini; 1993. p. 249–54.
14. Homoe P, Bretlau P. Cholesteatomas in the greenlandic inuit. In: Nakano Y, editor. Proceedings of the Fourth International Conference on cholesteatoma and mastoid surgery, Niigata, Japan. Amsterdam: Kugel & Gehdini; 1993. p. 241–4.

15. Tschopp C. Chronic otitis media and cholesteatoma in Alaskan children. In: McCabe B, Sade J, Abramson M, editors. Cholesteatoma: first international conference. Birmingham: Aesculapius Publishing Company; 1977. p. 290–2.
16. Tos M, Thomsen J, Peitersen E. Proceeding of the Third International Conference on cholesteatoma and mastoid surgery. Amsterdam: Kugel & Gehdini; 1989.
17. Deguine C, Deguine O. The contralateral ear in cholesteatoma. In: Tos M, Peitersen E, editors. Proceeding of the Third International Conference on cholesteatoma and mastoid surgery. Amsterdam: Kugel & Gehdini; 1989. p. 393–8.
18. Harell M, Pennigton FR, Morrison WV. Prevalence of cholesteatoma in Black Americans. In: Sade J, editor. Cholesteatoma and mastoid surgery. Amsterdam: Kugel & Gehdini; 1989. p. 97–9.
19. Ruben RJ. The disease in society—evaluation of chronic otitis media in general and cholesteatoma in particular. In: Sade J, editor. Cholesteatoma and mastoid surgery. Amsterdam: Kugel & Gehdini; 1989. p. 111–6.
20. Hildmann H, Steinbach E. Zur Wiedervervendung des autologen Ambosses beim Cholesteatoma und bei der chronischen Schleimhauteiterung. Laryngol-Rnhinol-Otol. 1972;51:659–60.
21. Frese KA, Hoppe F. Morphorlogische Untersuchungen an autologen und homologen Ossikeln nach Langzeitimplantation. Laryngol-Rnhinol-Otol. 1996;75:330–4.
22. Helms J. Sanierende und rekostruktive Operationen am Gehoergang, Mittelohr und Felsenbein.in Kopf und Hals-Chirurgie. Band 2:Ohr. J. Helms; R.A. Jahrsdoerfer. New York: Georg Thieme Verlag Stuttgart; 1996. p. 67–130.

5 Perioperative Issues Related to Cochlear Implantation

Hongwei Zheng, Jiahui Zhou, and Lisheng Yu

More than 800,000 people with severe hearing loss have received a cochlear implant and have returned to the world of sound. Since the introduction of the cochlear implant, with the deepening of people's understanding of the physiology and pathology of hearing and the improvement of precision technology, cochlear implant hardware and software technology has been constantly breaking through, so that the cochlear implantation surgery for the protection of the inner ear tissue structure and the reconstruction of the fine structure of the sound level has been significantly improved. The implantation concept is constantly being updated, the adapted population is expanding, and the sound reconstruction is improving day by day. Along with the large number of implantation surgeries, there has been a great deal of attention paid to the updating of implantation-related tests and examinations, the selection of indications for cochlear implantation, and the surgical paths and techniques for implantation.

5.1 Preoperative Examination for Cochlear Implantation

Currently, cochlear implantation is feasible for more than 90% of patients with severe sensorineural hearing loss. With the improvement of technology, the indications for surgery have been gradually relaxed, for example, the hearing standard for cochlear implantation in the United States has been relaxed from 75 dB in the bare ear in the past to 70 dB at present; some patients with auditory neuropathy have also achieved satisfactory results after cochlear implantation. However, there are still a few patients who are not suitable for cochlear implantation and should be checked as much as possible before surgery. The preoperative examination includes many elements, the most important of which are audiologic and imaging examinations.

5.1.1 Audiological Examination

The primary goal is to find out if the child has an auditory response. If there is an auditory response, the auditory pathway is often intact and cochlear implantation is usually feasible (except in rare cases of central lesions). If there is no auditory response at all, further investigations such as 40 Hz auditory event-related potential, audio steady-state response, electrical stimulation of the tympanic promontory, E-ABR, etc. are

H. Zheng · J. Zhou · L. Yu (✉)
Department of Otorhinolaryngology, Head and Neck Surgery, People's Hospital, Peking University, Beijing, China
e-mail: zhenghongwei@pku.edu.cn

L. Yu (ed.), *Progress in Postauricular Administration*, Experts' Perspectives on Medical Advances,
https://doi.org/10.1007/978-981-95-5102-6_5

needed. The response to strong acoustic stimuli can be observed after the child is allowed to wear a high-power hearing aid. In patients without residual hearing, pure tone audiometry, acoustic field audiometry, 40 Hz auditory event-related potential, audio steady-state response, etc. cannot truly reflect the residual function of the patient's auditory nerve, and the integrity of the auditory pathway can be predicted preoperatively by electrical stimulation of the drum cape, which can be used as a basis for cochlear implantation. In 1974, House et al. first used electrical stimulation of the drum cape to assess the electrical response of surviving spiral ganglion nerve fibers in patients with cochlear implantation and to predict postoperative auditory perception preoperatively [1]. Bento et al. used electrical stimulation of the drum cape to assess the integrity of the auditory pathway after resection of a type 2 acoustic neuroma [2]. Silverstein et al. concluded that the results of electrical stimulation of the drum cape reflected the number of cochlear remnants of the spiral ganglion [3]. Kuo et al. analyzed 290 patients with preoperative electrical stimulation of the drum capsule. Eighty-nine percent of the patients who responded to electrical stimulation gained hearing postoperatively (speech discrimination score of 70–95%) and concluded that the postoperative speech recognition rate after cochlear implantation was significantly correlated with the results of preoperative electrical stimulation of the drum capsule; in particular patients who had a better ability to discriminate the frequency in the drum capsule electrical stimulation (about 80%) had a significantly better postoperative open-item speech discrimination score than those who had a poorer ability to discriminate the frequency in the drum capsule electrical stimulation (about 70%) [4].

5.1.2 Imageological Examination

At present, the imaging diagnosis of inner ear malformation mainly relies on high-resolution CT and MRI. CT can clearly show the structure of the osseous labyrinth and understand the development of the cochlea in the temporal bone (whether it is normal or not and whether there is any deformity), the condition of the internal auditory canal (whether there is any narrowing of the internal auditory canal or any loss of the floor of the internal auditory canal), the anatomical variations (whether the ethmoidal sinus is shifted anteriorly or not, whether the jugular bulb is elevated or not, and whether the facial nerve is in the course of the facial nerve), the situation of the airiness of mastoid, and the presence of underlying otitis media or cholesteatoma. The use of MRI for preoperative examination of cochlear implantation is becoming more widespread with the improvement of imaging techniques. Compared with HRCT, MRI, especially water imaging of the inner ear, can not only clearly observe the structure of the inner ear membrane labyrinth but also show the development of the auditory nerve, which provides rich and reliable imaging information for the preoperative evaluation of cochlear implantation in children with congenital inner ear developmental malformations. Studies have shown that the water imaging sequence of MRI can visualize the structure of the membranous labyrinth by displaying the morphologic distribution and signal characteristics of the integrated image of the internal and external lymphatic fluid contained in the osseous labyrinth system and understand the development of the auditory nerve through the high signal background of the cerebrospinal fluid of the internal auditory canal and the pontine cerebellar angle area in contrast to the iso-low signal of the nerve within the internal auditory canal, which is of irreplaceable advantage in judging the inner ear labyrinth malformations and their classification and degree. It has an irreplaceable advantage in determining the classification and degree of inner ear labyrinth malformations. At the same time, MRI-based preoperative imaging diagnosis of cochlear implantation in patients with inner ear malformations can provide a reliable basis for the formulation of surgical plans, the selection of appropriate cochlear implant devices and electrodes, and the prediction of possible intraoperative situations. MRI is mainly used for patients with suspected ossification of the labyrinth (history of meningitis, otosclerosis), complete lack of response to various audiological examinations, and patients who do not have any postcochlear lesions. MRI is recommended before cochlear surgery in adults.

5.2 Selection of Indications for Cochlear Implantation

5.2.1 Cochlear Implantation in Younger Children

Due to the presence of a language plasticity period, younger children with profound deafness have always had the greatest benefit from cochlear implantation. Currently, the age of implantation is decreasing. The youngest reported age for implantation is even 3–4 months. Studies have shown that up to 3 years of age is a critical period for auditory-verbal development, and early cochlear implantation can expose children to auditory-verbal environments as early as possible, enhancing language skills, quality of speech, and expanding expressive and receptive vocabulary. Numerous studies have shown that auditory-verbal recovery is better in patients with cochlear implants before the age of 2 years and preferably before the age of 1 year. The literature shows that children with cochlear implants within 12 months of age achieve full development of hearing and speech skills. Auditory function tests such as behavioral audiometry, otoacoustic emissions, frequency-specific auditory brainstem response (ABR), or multifrequency steady-state response (ASSR) for younger children, as well as refined imaging such as MRI and endoauditory canal hydrography, enable reliable early diagnosis, the latter of which is critical for cochlear implantation in children younger than 12 months; several cochlear implant groups have reported that anesthesia and surgery are safe for children between the ages of 7 and 12 months. Anesthesia and surgery are safe in children aged 7–12 months. A study by Thompson et al. (48 implantations less than 18 months old, including 21 implantations less than 1 year old) showed that younger children with cochlear implantation had better hearing and speech after follow-up investigations [5]. Several studies by Roland et al. have confirmed that the rate of surgical complications in cochlear implantation in children younger than 12 months old is not significantly different from that in older children and in the adult group. The cochlear implantation rate in children younger than 12 months old is not significantly different from that of older children (Roland et al.) [6].

5.2.2 Cochlear Implantation in the Presence of Inner Ear Malformations

Inner ear malformations have more criteria for their classification; initially in 1987, Jackler et al. proposed a classification based on embryological and radiological studies, which categorized inner ear malformations into Michel's malformation, common cavity malformations, cochlear failure, cochlear hypoplasia, and Mondini's malformation; and in 2013, Sennaroglu et al. proposed a new classification method for inner ear malformations. He categorized inner ear malformations into the following types:

(1) Michel's malformation, the cochlea and vestibular structures are completely missing.
(2) Initial auditory vesicle; incomplete development of the auditory capsule, no internal auditory canal, between the Michel's malformation and the common cavity.
(3) Cochlea is underdeveloped; the cochlea is completely missing.
(4) The common cavity is malformed, the cochlea and vestibule fused into a capsule cavity, and there is no separation between the two.
(5) Cochlea is underdeveloped, the deformity is further polarized, and the cochlea and the vestibule are separated, but the underdevelopment is smaller than normal, resembling a small vesicle at the inner auditory canal. However, the cochlea and vestibule are smaller than normal, and the underdeveloped cochlea resembles a small vesicle in the inner auditory canal.

(6) Incomplete partition (IP): IP-I, in which the cochlea lacks all of the cochlear axis and the sieve region, and the cochlea is saccate with an enlarged cystic vestibule; IP-II, Mondini's malformation, in which the cochlea is only 1.5 weeks long, with the middle and parietal circumferences fused to form a cystic apex; IP-III, in which there is a septum but no cochlear axis, and the floor of the internal auditory canal is enlarged and communicates with the cochlear floor gyrus. In type IP-II, Mondini's malformation, the cochlea is only 1.5 weeks, the middle periphery and the top periphery are fused to form a cystic apex, accompanied by an enlarged vestibular aqueduct; IP-III, the cochlea has a septum but no cochlear axis, and the base of the internal auditory canal is dilated and communicates with the cochlear base gyrus; this is a kind of X-linked hereditary deafness, which is prone to "blowout" during cochlear implantation. This is a type of X-linked genetic deafness and is prone to "blowout" during cochlear implantation. If blowout occurs during the operation, the posterior arch column needs to be removed, the anvil and stapes bone need to be removed, and large muscles need to be used for vestibular tamponade. Intraoperative facial nerve monitoring is required;
(7) Large vestibular aqueduct syndrome.
(8) Abnormal development of the cochlear aperture; in addition, there are vestibular malformations, malformations of the internal auditory canal, and hemianopic malformations. Currently, with the exception of labyrinthine defects, initial auditory vesicles, and undeveloped cochlea, cochlear implantation can be performed in most patients with cochlear malformations through adequate preoperative evaluation and the use of electrodes of the appropriate length and type and can achieve more favorable results. It should be noted that for cochlear implantation in patients with inner ear malformations, accurate preoperative evaluation and intraoperative CT real-time guidance are important in guiding the path of electrode insertion, determining the position of the electrode in real time, and avoiding surgical complications in individual patients with malformations of the middle ear and inner ear structures, especially in patients with facial nerve location, severe malformations of the cochlear structure, and traffic between the internal auditory canal and the cochlea. In patients with certain inner ear malformations, such as common cavity malformations and cochlear developmental insufficiency, care should be taken not to force the cochlear electrode to be implanted in its entirety, so as not to mistakenly enter the inner auditory canal and cause serious postoperative complications. Stenosis of the internal auditory canal and underdevelopment of the auditory nerve should also be carefully evaluated. Literature shows that as long as the auditory nerve has about 30% of nerve fibers, cochlear implantation can achieve good results. If the patient has a preoperative auditory response (preferably after wearing a hearing aid) or a response to E-ABR, cochlear implantation can mostly be performed.

5.2.3 Cochlear Implantation for Auditory Neuropathy

Auditory neuropathy (AN) is a group of auditory disorders in which the auditory brainstem evoked response is not elicited and the otoacoustic emissions are normal, with impaired speech comprehension as the main manifestation. In recent years, it is also known as auditory neuropathy spectrum disorder, which was first named by Starr et al. in 1996 [7]. From the analysis of electrophysiological findings, the auditory neuropathy is a postcochlear lesion, and the patient's outer hair cell function is normal, and the site of the lesion is most likely to be located between the inner hair cell and the brainstem, that is, any inner hair cell, spiral ganglion, connection between the inner hair cells and synapses, the axon of auditory nerves, or its branches, and the auditory pathway of the brainstem may be the site of the lesion in an auditory neuropathy. The lesion affects the ability to process sound signals, which are not transmitted synchronously. Etiologic studies have suggested that the disease is divided into nongenetic and genetic factors. The main clinical interventions for AN include medication, hearing aids, and cochlear implants.

Early on, auditory neuropathy was considered to be a purely auditory nerve dysfunction such as demyelination resulting in desynchronization of nerve conduction and was therefore listed as a contraindication to cochlear implantation. In the late 1990s, Miyamoto and Rance et al. were the first to report that a small sample of patients with auditory neuropathy experienced varying degrees of improvement in their hearing thresholds and speech recognition after attempting to implant a cochlear implant [8, 9]. Shallop et al. improved both speech perception thresholds and speech reception thresholds after cochlear implantation in five children with AN, who were unable to discriminate speech before cochlear implantation and gained the ability to discriminate words after surgery [10]. Zeng et al. showed that speech recognition scores of cochlear implanted patients with auditory neuropathy could reach the average level of non-AN cochlear implant recipients [11]. As reported by Raveh et al., 12 children with AN who received cochlear implants had better outcomes, and some had improved speech production [12]. Gibson et al. reported that 75% of 60 patients with AN had speech recognition scores that were comparable to those of control patients with SNHL (sensorineural hearing loss) [13]. Fulmer et al. found that monosyllabic and bisyllabic word speech recognition scores in quiet and noise conditions in both the acoustic neuropathy and sensorineural deafness groups after cochlear implantation were higher than those of patients with SNHL, and two-syllable word speech recognition scores in quiet and noise conditions [14]. It is clear that cochlear implantation can provide good speech discrimination for sensorineural deaf patients and is the only clinically proven treatment that may be effective for AN. However, not all patients with AN can be rehabilitated by cochlear implantation, and Bradley et al. reported that cochlear implantation was not effective in patients with AN who had auditory nerve hypoplasia or agnosia [15]. Walton et al. reported poor results of cochlear implantation in patients with peripheral neuropathy, especially in a subset of syndromic AN [16]. Zdanski et al. reported the results of cochlear implantation in a child with unexplained peripheral neurologic symptoms starting at age 2 years, and at 18 months postoperatively, the child's open-item monosyllabic word recognition scores were not significantly different from those of the preoperative period and the intraoperative and postoperative failure to elicit ECAP , suggesting that cochlear implantation did not serve to restore synchronization of neural activity in this patient [17]. It is also worth noting that a significant proportion of patients with AN who do not have abnormalities of auditory nerve development and other peripheral neuropathies still have a high degree of individual variability in the outcome of cochlear implantation and are difficult to anticipate on the basis of preoperative clinical performance. Theoretically, if the AN lesion is in the inner hair cell or synapse, the cochlear implant can bypass this part of the afferent pathway and stimulate the auditory neuron cell or axon directly; if the lesion is in the auditory nerve trunk, cochlear stimulation can improve or partially improve the problem of auditory neural desynchronization due to better synchronization of electrical signals; and if the mechanism of the lesion is the neuron loss, the cochlear implantation will be ineffective. However, since there is no diagnostic method to accurately identify the different subtypes of AN lesions, the effect of cochlear implantation can only be indirectly predicted by the clinical manifestations before surgery. It is clear that cochlear implantation in patients with AN involving peripheral neuropathy and imaging evidence of abnormal development or absence of the auditory nerve is not effective. It is highly unlikely that such patients will achieve the cochlear implant results of the average SNHL patient. Similarly in patients with syndromic auditory neuropathies such as Leber's optic neuropathy, Stevens-Johnson syndrome (mucocutaneous syndrome),

Ehlers-Danlos syndrome (congenital connective tissue hypoplasia syndrome), progressive peroneal muscular dystrophy (Charcot-Marie-Tooth (CMT) disease), and deafness-dystonia-optic neuronopathy syndrome, cochlear implantation is not effective and should be implanted with caution.

5.2.4 Cochlear Implantation in Cerebral White Matter Lesions

With the widespread development of MRI, the diagnosis of cerebral white matter lesions has increased significantly in recent years. Some of them are caused by genetic or biochemical mechanisms and belong to the category of cerebral white matter dystrophy, while others are caused by nongenetic acquired factors such as immunity, inflammation, and environment and belong to cerebral white matter demyelination. Leukodystrophy can progressively worsen with age and can lead to movement disorders, mental retardation, speech disorders, etc., while some patients have slow progression of the disease or have no clinical symptoms. Lapointe et al. showed that 20% of patients with profound bilateral deafness had significant brain abnormalities on MRI and that leukodystrophy was the most common type of leukodystrophy, accounting for 70% of patients [18]. This may be related to brain injuries such as infection, ischemia, hypoxia, or prematurity before and after birth, as well as abnormalities of the white matter myelin sheath caused by genetics or immune, inflammatory, and environmental factors. At the same time, some children with abnormal white matter development can achieve the same level of hearing and speech recovery after cochlear implantation as prelingually deaf children without white matter lesions through regular rehabilitation training. Luthra et al. summarized the evaluation of the effect of cochlear implantation in five cases of deaf children with combined white matter abnormalities and found that compared with deaf children with normal white matter, deaf children with abnormalities of the white matter had varying degrees of hearing and speech recovery after implantation. The hearing and speech recovery was impaired. In Moon et al.'s study, the behavioral scores of hearing and speech rehabilitation of children with white matter lesions differed from those of the control group at 6 months after cochlear implantation, but there was no significant difference at 1 year after the operation [19]. After cochlear implantation in prelingually deaf children with mild white matter anomalies and after regular rehabilitation training, there was no significant difference in the effect of hearing and speech rehabilitation between these children and those who had no syndromes or obvious etiologies of prelingually deaf children. In view of the uncertainty of the effect of white matter lesions on the postoperative rehabilitation effect of cochlear implantation, with the deepening of the study, white matter disease, especially stable white matter lesions, is no longer a contraindication for cochlear implantation.

5.2.5 Cochlear Implantation in the Presence of Inflammatory Lesions in the Middle Ear

Inflammatory lesions in the middle ear were once listed as a contraindication to cochlear implantation because of the presence of inflammatory lesions in the area where the electrode passes through, which may lead to inner ear infections and intracranial complications after the surgery. However, with the continuous development of clinical technology, cochlear implantation in patients with otitis media is gradually being developed. Chronic nonpurulent otitis media is not a contraindication to cochlear implantation, and cochlear implantation can be performed in stage I. Luntz et al. reported that 70.0% (7/10) of children with otitis media susceptible to otitis media and 37.5% (3/8) of normal children were found to have thickened edematous mucosa, and the cochlear window niches were often found to be obstructed by edematous mucous membranes, which had to be cleared in order to recognize the cochlear window niches [20]. It has been reported in the literature that the frequency and severity of otitis media in children with otitis media do not increase after cochlear implantation and that conventional antibiotic therapy can effectively control the disease. Fayad et al. retrospectively found that among 61 children with otitis media who were successfully followed up, 78% had a decreased frequency of otitis media after surgery, 19% had no change, and 3% had an increased frequency, of which 11 tympanic tube patients had a decreased frequency of otitis media after surgery, without any infectious complication [21]. The frequency of otitis media decreased in all 11 cases of tympanic tube placement without any infectious complications, and therefore cochlear implantation in children with nonpurulent otitis media is considered safe. For children with suppurative otitis media that is not effectively controlled, cochlear implantation is generally considered a contraindication. A two-stage procedure is often required. One-stage surgery begins with management of the purulent inflammatory lesion. However, Colletti et al. suggested that if the patient has persistent chronic suppurative otitis media, the middle cranial fossa approach can be used to implant electrodes at the base of the middle cranial fossa for the cochlear base gyrus, which has the advantage of avoiding otogenic infection by not passing through the infected mastoid cavity of the middle ear but increases the risk associated with craniotomy [22]. For those with tympanic membrane perforation as a sequela of otitis media, if the tympanic mucosa is dry and there is no inflammation, adult patients can choose stage I tympanic membrane repair + cochlear implantation or staged surgery; pediatric patients may have poor Eustachian tube function, and other factors, in principle, should be staged surgery. For middle ear cholesteatoma, one-stage or two-stage surgery can be chosen according to the patient's condition. Patients who have undergone radical mastoidectomy and are proposed to undergo cochlear implantation should preferably undergo staged surgery, with one-stage surgery to close the surgical cavity and two-stage surgery to implant the cochlear implant.

5.2.6 Bilateral Cochlear Implantation

In 1996, Jan Helm performed the first bilateral cochlear implant (BCI) in an adult and detected improvements in speech comprehension and directional hearing in this patient at 4 weeks postoperatively; BCIs were successfully applied to children in 1998. As of 2016, the total number of CIs worldwide amounted to more than 800,000, of which more than 70,000 were BCIs. Patients undergoing BCI have greater benefits in postoperative auditory-verbal rehabilitation and protection of the auditory center. BCI patients have been shown to have better speech recognition and sound localization. Smulders et al. conducted a multicenter randomized clinical trial that showed that BCIs localized sound significantly better than a unilateral cochlear implant group, which was consistent with self-assessment of subjects' hearing ability [23]. Coez et al. used electron emission computed tomography (EECT) to examine the benefits of BCIs compared to unilateral implants. Compared to unilateral implantation, BCI enhanced spectral cues associated with sound perception and improved processing of speech stimuli in the right temporal region; it also resulted in enhanced sound discrimination by recruiting sensory information in the right frontoparietal network [24]. Patients who underwent BCI had greater benefits in terms of postoperative auditory-verbal rehabilitation and preservation of the auditory center. Lee et al. showed that BCI lowered mean hearing thresholds by 7.2–7.4 dB compared with UCI. Lovett et al. showed that sound source localization was improved by 18.5%, and speech recognition in noisy environments was improved by 20% after BCI [25]. Meanwhile, although BCI technology has become more mature and has clear efficacy, implanted individuals still have certain deficits compared to normal individuals. Most studies have found that the binaural benefits of BCI implant recipients hardly approach those of normal individuals, and a study by Reiss et al. found extensive abnormal fusion of binaural tones in bilateral cochlear implant users [26]. Although slightly wider binaural fusion may be beneficial for sound localization, it has been shown that extremely wide fusion of octave scales can interfere with speech perception, especially when there is a large interaural pitch mismatch. Also, binaural benefits are limited by cochlear devices, coding strategies, and other limitations. For bilateral implantation in infants, the surgery should not take too long and should be performed by an experienced surgeon. Intraoperative bleeding should also be minimized.

5.3 Problems Associated with Implantation Surgery

5.3.1 Selection of the Implantation Side

Ninety-eight percent of right-handed individuals rely primarily on the left cerebral hemisphere to process language, whereas the majority of left-handed individuals (approximately 60%) also rely primarily on the left hemisphere (Risse et al. 1997) [27]. Since left-handed individuals make up only 7–8% of the total population, this means that 96% of individuals in the total population process language with a left hemisphere-specific feature that is independent of the individual's sharp hand. Therefore, if the situation is similar bilaterally, the right implant is preferred.

5.3.2 Choice of Access for Implantation Surgery

Currently, the main surgical approaches for cochlear implantation are:

(1) Nerve crypt approach behind the ear: the most commonly used surgical approach for cochlear implantation, mainly through the cochleostomy or through the membrane of the round window to implant the electrodes, the method provides better visualization and exposure of the round window, which helps the electrode arrays to be inserted and retained, and the mastoid is opened to ensure that the surgery has a good field of view, the cochlear window is fully exposed, and the direction of electrode implantation is closer to the drum step alignment, which is conducive to the delivery of the electrodes. The direction of electrode implantation is close to the drum step, which is favorable for electrode delivery. At the same time, the larger space of the mastoid cavity can be used to place the electrode wires of rich length, which ensures that the electrode tension is maintained in a small state after the operation, and there is no surgical operation on the tympanic membrane and the external auditory canal, so that their normal physiological functions are preserved, and the structural normality of the middle ear is maintained to the maximum extent, and the residual hearing is preserved in the patient. The key point is to fully expose the tympanic sinus and identify the anvil body. This mostly allows visualization of the horizontal segment of the facial nerve, and the plane of the vertical segment can be roughly surmised. The saphenous approach also has some limitations: due to the small operating space at the saphenous fossa, there is the possibility of injury to the facial nerve and/or the tympanic cord. Hoffman reported that the incidence of facial paralysis was as high as 0.56% in adults and 0.27% in children [28]. In patients with cochlear ossification, the ossification is usually located at the beginning of the cochlear base turn, which prevents smooth implantation of the electrodes and may lead to electrode damage. In addition, in patients with acute and chronic middle ear infections and after radical mastoidectomy, complex preparatory and restorative surgery is required to avoid implanting the electrode into the infected area, which may lead to labyrinthitis and secondary meningitis, thus increasing the difficulty of performing this procedure in these patients. Due to the limitation of the cochlear spiral structure, the implanted electrodes can only reach the cochlear base or a small portion of the cochlear mid-rotation, so

that the frequency signal of the implanted electrodes does not match the cochlear position.

(2) Superior external auditory canal approach: first proposed by Kronenberg in 1999, this approach greatly reduces the damage to the facial nerve by avoiding the open exposure of the facial nerve fossa [29]. The surgical operation of this technique is performed on the lateral side of the anvil bone, and the facial nerve is far away from the upper tunnel of the ear canal and is always under the protection of the anvil bone, so the damage to the facial nerve is almost zero, and although the tympanic nerve is exposed, the probability of damage is extremely small, and at the same time, by peeling off the posterior wall of the external auditory canal to reveal the middle tympanic chamber, the tympanic cape is exposed adequately, and the cochlear window can be clearly localized, so this approach is more suitable for patients with ossification of the cochlea. This route is more suitable for patients with cochlear ossification and can accurately locate the window of cochlear ossification. However, because of the need to separate the bone-tram flap of the external auditory canal, the incidence of skin tearing and tympanic membrane perforation of the external auditory canal is greatly increased, and there are problems with postoperative medication changes and ear canal tamponade in pediatric patients, and the difficulty of this procedure is dramatically increased for low-site dura mater, which is why Kronenberg et al. concluded that low-site dura mater is a contraindication to this procedure.

(3) The middle cranial fossa pathway was first reported by Colletti in 1998, broadening the surgical indications for cochlear implantation [22]. It is suitable for patients with bilateral mastoidectomy, chronic middle ear disease, middle and inner ear malformations, and partial ossification of the cochlear base, and because of the accurate electrode position, the patient's postoperative speech perception is significantly improved. However, this approach is time-consuming, and Colletti et al. reported that the duration of surgery using this approach was 2–3 h, which was significantly higher than the previous two procedures, and there was a risk of serious intracranial complications. There is a risk of injury to the temporal lobe, middle meningeal artery, and other neurovascular vessels when stripping the dura mater. Because it is a craniotomy, the patient's family and the surgeon will be under greater psychological pressure, and most otolaryngologists are unfamiliar with the structure of the middle cranial fossa, and the lack of experience in craniotomy also restricts the popularization and application of this type of surgery.

(4) Minimally invasive approach and robot-assisted minimally invasive approach: with the development of science and technology as well as the research and practice of minimally invasive surgery, minimally invasive approach can better preserve the patient's original residual hearing, and at the same time, it has the advantages of less trauma, fewer surgical complications, and aesthetics. However, the operative field is narrower, which leads to more difficult surgery and requires more anatomical knowledge and surgical skills of the surgeon. In 2017, the robotic system was successfully applied for the first time and clinical trials were carried out [30]. The precision of the robotic drilling is 0.2 mm, and its safety mechanism can predict the nerve within 0.1 mm. The cochlear electrode was successfully inserted into the robotic drilling tunnel through the smallest incision without any postoperative complications, and at the same time, it has also excellent preservation of surrounding structures. With the improvement of the robotic cochlear implantation system and its workflow, the clinical application of this surgical method is feasible. In the author's experience, various surgical accesses for cochlear implantation have served for successful implantation, and the choice of the specific surgical access should be based on a rigorous evaluation of the patient's condition, as well as a compre-

hensive analysis of the social, psychological, and economic factors and the surgeon's condition, in order to select the optimal surgical approach.

5.3.3 "Clean" Minimally Invasive Surgery

In 1993, Lehnhardt proposed the so-called soft-surgery technique, which takes into account the damage to the cochlea during cochlear implantation surgery and suggests how to minimally invade the cochlea [31], and in 2002, O'Donoghue and Nikolo-poulos proposed a small-incision, minimally invasive technique for the Nucleus24 technique [32]. It is important to note that minimally invasive implantation is a relative concept, in contrast to previous conventional CI surgery, in which unnecessary injuries are minimized or avoided, with the goal of keeping the incision as small and aesthetically pleasing as possible, localizing the scalp at the implant site, preserving the fine structure of the cochlea and its internal environment, maximizing the preservation of residual hearing, preventing flap complications and electrode migration, and providing for the possibility of reimplantation of the CI, future acceptance of the CI, stem cell transplantation, hair cell regeneration, and deaf implantation. It also preserves the conditions for possible CI reimplantation, future treatment with new technologies such as stem cell transplantation, hair cell regeneration, and gene therapy for deafness. It is important to note that a simple small incision is not the same as noninvasive. In the author's opinion, the appropriate surgical incision needs to be rigorously designed and considered and should not be pursued as a small incision, especially for beginners. The cochlear implantation incision needs to consider the postoperative speech processor wear and the patient's anatomy. It is important to avoid scarring of the incision that may affect the use of the cochlear implant. At the same time, too small an incision will increase the degree of intraoperative pulling on the flap. Excessive pulling will cause edema of the flap, which may result in difficulty in healing the flap, and scarring will increase the electrical resistance and decrease the dynamic range of the cochlea. Minimally invasive surgical design should give due consideration to aesthetics, avoidance of complications, increased surgical safety, preservation of cochlear microstructure, preservation of residual hearing, and prevention of cochlear fibrosis. The author's experience suggests that appropriate incision and flap design can effectively minimize flap complications, avoid or minimize damage to the middle ear tympanic membrane and auditory ossicular chain as well as cochlear microstructures, aggressively and thoroughly ensure hemostasis, and avoid an overly deep bone groove for placement of the implant. An overly deep bone slot requires exposure of a large area of the dura mater so that the appearance is smooth and the implant does not protrude from the bone surface. However, this has the consequence that the cranium loses its bony protection, and in the event of trauma to the area, the cranium can be easily damaged, and there may be a fatal risk of an epidural hematoma. And it will make the skin flap relatively thick, increase the resistance, reduce the dynamic range, and affect the use. With the appropriate depth of the bone groove, although the implant may appear to be elevated, the skin flap has a certain degree of tension, and there is a so-called tight pocket effect, which can effectively avoid postoperative edema of the skin flap and subcutaneous accumulation of blood and fluid. At the same time to avoid the destruction of the cochlear microstructure, during the operation, hormone and sodium hyaluronate can be applied simultaneously to protect the inner ear function and cochlear environment, effectively preventing inflammation, fibrosis, or ossification of the cochlea and preserving the necessary cochlear conditions for possible future high-tech treatments—stem cell transplantation, hair cell regeneration, and gene therapy for deafness. Generally speaking, there are traumatic injuries on the way to cochlear implantation, such as skin, periosteum, mastoid process, implant bone groove, and cochlear window opening, except that the operators are aware of this problem and are now considering to minimize the trauma as much as possible. Instead of overly pursuing small incisions and minimally invasive surgery, the author believes that "clean surgery" is more important. The so-called clean surgery should be carried out throughout the entire cochlear implantation surgery, including the production of appropriate skin flap and myoperiosteal flap, thorough hemostasis and cleaning of the surgical cavity, proper implant fixation, accurate window opening, and electrode implantation. Appropriate flap and flap creation refers to the use of slightly different surgical incisions according to the patient's head condition and the shape of different implants, avoiding too small an incision. The design of the incision and the flap should take into account the position of the postauricular pendant and the transmission coil to ensure easy use of the cochlear implant. Care should be taken to avoid a low incision that may result in scarring of the incision affecting the use of the cochlear implant. Webb et al. studied 712 cochlear implant surgeries and found that the most significant complication was incision nonhealing, with 0.6–2.0% of patients requiring removal of the implant [33]. Cohen pointed out that most of the complications were related to the anterior C-shaped flap at the base, emphasizing that the flap design and size are very important and that the flap must be sufficiently large, with an incision that is away from the implant, and should be sutured tension-free and that the lower limb of the C-shaped flap may cut off the blood supply from the posterior ear artery if the flap extends beyond the lower edge of the earlobe [34]. If the lower limb of the C-shaped flap extends beyond the lower edge of the earlobe, it may cut off the flap's blood supply from the posterior auricular artery. In obese patients, especially adult patients, the musculoskeletal flap is thinned, and it should usually be no more than approximately 6 mm thick to reduce electrical resistance and increase the dynamic range of the cochlear implant. Care needs to be taken throughout the procedure to ensure thorough hemostasis and cleanliness of the operative cavity, especially in infant patients, to adequately stop bleeding and minimize blood loss. Attention should be paid to the process of separating the musculoskeletal flap to avoid unclear layers and mistakenly entering the muscle layer, which can easily cause postoperative blood accumulation under the flap and affect the healing of the flap. Avoiding inadequate hemostasis is crucial, as it can cause flap hematoma and potentially necessitate a second surgery. And once the cochlear implant is installed, only bipolar electrocoagulation can be used; electric knife cannot be used. Intraoperative care should be taken to stop bleeding thoroughly, small clots within the tympanic cavity can affect the opening of the tympanic capsule or exposure of the round window membrane, and the cavity must be thoroughly cleaned before implanting the electrodes, especially the broken bone fragments. Bone fragments attached to the electrode may cause implantation difficulties. Note that blood and bone dust in the cavity may cause postoperative adhesions and fibrous growths, which may also make reimplantation more difficult. For proper implant fixation, it is important not to place the implant too deeply into the bone groove to avoid exposing a large area of the dura mater, and a thin layer of bone outside the dura mater can avoid these problems. Experienced doctors with short surgery times can use small incisions. However, small incisions are not recommended for surgeons with a long operating time. In addition to poor exposure, prolonged pulling on the flap may lead to edema of the flap, which may affect healing. And if fibrosis occurs after edema, it will thicken the flap, increase the resistance, and reduce the dynamic range. And poor fixation and slippage of the implant may result in implant failure and the need to replace the implant again. In the case of a small mastoid with a markedly anterior displacement of the sigmoid sinus, a pendulous canopy, or a severely sclerotic mastoid, the external auditory canal flap can be lifted and the round window positioned for cochlear implantation. Ear cartilage is then removed to reconstruct the posterior wall of the external auditory canal to protect the electrode. Accurate electrode implantation involves precise localization of the window opening, especially in patients with cochlear deformities. Note that the cochlear opening is usually located in the upper part of the round window niche. The cochlear windowing is performed by following the extension of the long peduncle axis of the anvil bone and spacing the cochlear windowing at a distance of one stapes head medial to the long protrusion of the anvil bone. In children and in patients with inner ear malformations, sometimes the cochlea rotates superiorly or medially, and sometimes the oval and round windows undergo significant variations, making surgical manipulation significantly more difficult. If the cochlear window is inappropriately located, it can cause the illusion of ossification. If continued outward grinding cannot enter the cavity of the cochlear basal gyrus, and if drilling too deeply may reach the high jugular bulb or internal carotid artery, especially in younger children, the position of the facial nerve is relatively high, and the cochlea may also be rotated forward and upward, and the direction of the window opening should be biased toward the medial side and upward, and it is sometimes necessary to enlarge the surgical scope. Care should be taken to avoid opening too far forward, opening the internal carotid canal, or opening too far up, opening between the basal and second gyrus, or opening the second gyrus. Care is also taken to open the window perpendicular to the cochlea to avoid crossing the round window niche and entering the inferior tympanic cavity. In addition, the window is too large and the use of soft tissue closure may make reoperation more difficult. When opening the cochlea, it is important to observe the condition of the external lymphatic cavity; if you grind the head of the drum too far down, sometimes the illusion of long-distance ossification is created (in fact, the external lymphatic cavity is normal), and this does not allow you to open the cochlea. With overpneumatization, sometimes the electrode can mistakenly pass below the basal gyrus and into the pneumatic chamber. Ossification of the cochlea is most often seen in patients with purulent meningitis or otosclerosis, and the sclerotic foci of intralesional otosclerosis can mostly be carefully removed with a small crochet hook. Sclerotic foci after purulent meningitis are very dense and can only be removed by abrasion. If necessary, a second return needs to be opened for implantation. Before electrode implantation, it is important to clean the operative cavity, remove fine bone debris, and stop bleeding adequately; electrodes with attached bone debris may make implantation difficult. The implantation process needs to be precise and slow, gently pushing the electrode into the cochlea. Too rapid implantation may cause air bubbles to appear in the cochlea, which may not be favorable for implantation. Note that rough or repeated insertion may result in short-circuiting of some electrodes. For models with reference electrodes, be sure to place the reference electrode under the periosteum. Placing the reference electrode inside the muscle will cause damage to the reference electrode due to repeated pulling by muscle contraction, and reimplantation is often required. Note that adult patients often do not require additional fixation of the stimulating electrode. In children, the size of the inner and middle ear is already similar to that of adults, but the mastoid process will expand outward by 1.5 cm with the growth of the skull, so it is necessary to fix the electrodes additionally, but care should be taken not to squeeze the electrodes unnecessarily. The extra electrode can be coiled inside the mastoid process. Generally there is no need to use other measures to seal the round window or the bulging cape opening, relying on the expansion of the electrode itself can often close the round window or the bulging cape opening, and if necessary, a small piece of muscle or connective tissue can be added. It is important to avoid the use of bone meal, otolithic gel, muscle or bone wax to fill the round window, cochlear aperture, and facial recesses during closure of the operative cavity or to hold the electrode in place in the mastoid process. These fillings can cause implantation difficulties when secondary cochlear implants are needed. Reoperation is risky and is recommended to be performed by an experienced surgeon. Care should be taken to close the incision layer by layer with absorbable sutures, avoiding the use of nonabsorbable sutures that can cause scarring. Also when closing the incision, improper handling, especially the suture needle used in suturing, may damage the electrodes and the implant, the implant loses its seal, and body fluids can enter, rendering the implant system ineffective.

In summary, cochlear implant hardware and software technology has been constantly breaking through, the implantation concept has been constantly updated, the applicable population has been constantly expanding, and sound reconstruction has been perfected day by day. As a result, the implantation-related testing and examination methods have been updated; the selection of indications for cochlear implantation and the implantation surgical pathway, surgical techniques, and other related issues are also changing day by day; and the criteria for the indications for cochlear implantation and the clinical practice have undergone significant changes, and early implantation of cochlear implantation no longer has a contraindication for cochlear implantation in children with prespeech deafness who have a good residual hearing at low frequencies and most of the cochlear deformities. The residual hearing is preserved, and acoustic-electricity is not a contraindication for cochlear implantation. Preservation of residual hearing, combined acoustic-electrical stimulation, and bilateral cochlear implantation are becoming more common. Improved surgical techniques and clean, minimally invasive procedures are reducing the need for cochlear implantation. There are still a large number of unanswered questions, but as time goes on and technology advances, more people will benefit from this technology.

References

1. House WF, Brackmann DE. Electrical promontory testing in differential diagnosis of sensori-neural hearing impairment. Laryngoscope. 1974;84(12):2163–71.
2. Bento RF, et al. Retrolabyrinthine approach for cochlear nerve preservation in neurofibromatosis type 2 and simultaneous cochlear implantation. Int Arch Otorhinolaryngol. 2013;17(3):351–5.
3. Silverstein H, et al. Promontory testing in neurotologic diagnosis. Am J Otolaryngol. 1994;15(1):101–7.
4. Kuo SC, Gibson WP. The role of the promontory stimulation test in cochlear implantation. Cochlear Implants Int. 2002;3(1):19–28.
5. Thompson DC, et al. Universal newborn hearing screening: summary of evidence. JAMA. 2001;286(16):2000–10.
6. Roland JT Jr, et al. Cochlear implantation in the very young child: long-term safety and efficacy. Laryngoscope. 2009;119(11):2205–10.
7. Starr A, et al. Auditory neuropathy. Brain. 1996;119(Pt 3):741–53.
8. Rance G, et al. Clinical findings for a group of infants and young children with auditory neuropathy. Ear Hear. 1999;20(3):238–52.
9. Miyamoto RT, et al. Cochlear implantation in auditory neuropathy. Laryngoscope. 1999;109(2 Pt 1):181–5.
10. Shallop JK, et al. Cochlear implants in five cases of auditory neuropathy: postoperative findings and progress. Laryngoscope. 2001;111(4 Pt 1):555–62.
11. Zeng FG, Liu S. Speech perception in individuals with auditory neuropathy. J Speech Lang Hear Res. 2006;49(2):367–80.
12. Raveh E, et al. Auditory neuropathy: clinical characteristics and therapeutic approach. Am J Otolaryngol. 2007;28(5):302–8.
13. Gibson WP, Graham JM. Editorial: 'auditory neuropathy' and cochlear implantation—myths and facts. Cochlear Implants Int. 2008;9(1):1–7.
14. Fulmer SL, et al. Rate of neural recovery in implanted children with auditory neuropathy spectrum disorder. Otolaryngol Head Neck Surg. 2011;144(2):274–9.
15. Bradley J, et al. Variable long-term outcomes from cochlear implantation in children with hypoplastic auditory nerves. Cochlear Implants Int. 2008;9(1):34–60.
16. Walton J, et al. Predicting cochlear implant outcomes in children with auditory neuropathy. Otol Neurotol. 2008;29(3):302–9.
17. Teagle HF, et al. Cochlear implantation in children with auditory neuropathy spectrum disorder. Ear Hear. 2010;31(3):325–35.
18. Lapointe A, et al. Central nervous system findings by magnetic resonance in children with profound sensorineural hearing loss. Int J Pediatr Otorhinolaryngol. 2006;70(5):863–8.
19. Moon IJ, et al. The clinical significance of preoperative brain magnetic resonance imaging in pediatric cochlear implant recipients. Audiol Neurootol. 2012;17(6):373–80.
20. Luntz M, Teszler CB, Shpak T. Cochlear implantation in children with otitis media: second stage of a long-term prospective study. Int J Pediatr Otorhinolaryngol. 2004;68(3):273–80.
21. Fayad JN, et al. Cochlear implantation in children with otitis media. Laryngoscope. 2003;113(7):1224–7.
22. Colletti V, et al. Basal turn cochleostomy via the middle fossa route for cochlear implant insertion. Am J Otolaryngol. 1998;19(6):778–84.
23. Smulders YE, et al. Comparison of bilateral and unilateral cochlear implantation in adults: a randomized clinical trial. JAMA Otolaryngol Head Neck Surg. 2016;142(3):249–56.
24. Coez A, et al. Brain voice processing with bilateral cochlear implants: a positron emission tomography study. Eur Arch Otorrinolaringol. 2014;271(12):3187–93.

25. Lovett RE, et al. Bilateral or unilateral cochlear implantation for deaf children: an observational study. Arch Dis Child. 2010;95(2):107–12.
26. Reiss LAJ, et al. Binaural pitch fusion in bilateral cochlear implant users. Ear Hear. 2018;39(2):390–7.
27. Risse GL, Gates JR, Fangman MC. A reconsideration of bilateral language representation based on the intracarotid amobarbital procedure. Brain Cogn. 1997;33(1):118–32.
28. Hoffman RA, Cohen NL. Complications of cochlear implant surgery. Ann Otol Kronenberg, J., L. Migirov, and T. Dagan, Suprameatal approach: new surgical approach for cochlear implantation. J Laryngol Otol. 2001;115(4):283–5.
29. Kronenberg J, Migirov L, Dagan T. Suprameatal approach: new surgical approach for cochlear implantation. J Laryngol Otol. 2001;115(4):283–5.
30. Caversaccio M, et al. Robotic cochlear implantation: surgical procedure and first clinical experience. Acta Otolaryngol. 2017;137(4):447–54.
31. Lehnhardt E. [Intracochlear placement of cochlear implant electrodes in soft surgery technique]. HNO. 1993;41(7):356–9.
32. O'Donoghue GM, Nikolopoulos TP. Minimal access surgery for pediatric cochlear implantation. Otol Neurotol. 2002;23(6):891–4.
33. Webb RL, et al. Surgical complications with the cochlear multiple-channel intracochlear implant: experience at Hannover and Melbourne. Ann Otol Rhinol Laryngol. 1991;100(2):131–6.
34. Cohen NL. Surgical techniques to avoid complications of cochlear implants in children. Adv Otorhinolaryngol. 1997;52:161–3.

6 Endolymphatic Sac Surgery for Meniere's Disease

Hongwei Zheng, Titi Pan, and Lisheng Yu

The primary goal of Ménière's disease treatment is to control the frequency of vertigo attacks, reduce the severity of vertigo episodes, minimize damage to auditory function, and improve hearing and tinnitus. Although surgical treatment of Meniere's disease remains controversial or questioned, several guidelines still include surgical treatment of Meniere's disease. Surgery remains a frequent and effective treatment option in our practice for patients who have failed conservative treatments or have poor outcomes. The usual surgical procedures include tympanic tube placement, endolymphatic sac decompression (truncation), semicircular canal tamponade, vestibular neurectomy, and vestibulectomy, among which endolymphatic sac decompression is the most commonly used surgical procedure, whereas destructive surgeries, including vestibular neurectomy, and vestibulectomy, have been less frequently used nowadays [1–3].

6.1 Endolymphatic Sac Decompression Surgery

Endolymphatic sac decompression was the most commonly performed surgical intervention in patients with Meniere's disease for a long time, but the necessity and effectiveness of the procedure remain controversial at this time. Portmann [4] first described endolymphatic sac decompression for the treatment of vertigo in 1927. Hallpike and Cairns [5] identified the pathological findings of endolymphatic effusion in patients with Meniere's disease in 1938, but by that time, the surgical approach described by Portmann was little used and reported from other otolaryngologists tended to pay less attention to the value of this approach. In 1962, William House [6] described good results with subarachnoid shunts for endolymphedema, which rekindled interest in this technique, but it was not until 1967 that kimura [7] reliably reproduced endolymphatic effusions in guinea pigs by destroying endolymphatic vessels and endolymphatic sacs that he provided some theoretical justification for this surgical approach. Since then, several interventions for endolymphatic sac effusions have been reported in several articles, including endolymphatic sac decompression, endolymphatic sac dissection, and endolymphatic sac drainage surgery [8–12]. Yokuta et al. also suggested the intraoperative glucocorticoid injection directly into the endolymphatic sac. These interventions

H. Zheng · T. Pan · L. Yu (✉)
Department of Otorhinolaryngology, Head and Neck Surgery, People's Hospital, Peking University, Beijing, China
e-mail: zhenghongwei@pku.edu.cn

L. Yu (ed.), *Progress in Postauricular Administration*, Experts' Perspectives on Medical Advances,
https://doi.org/10.1007/978-981-95-5102-6_6

are still suspected of having a nonspecific or placebo effect, despite the 60–95% success rate of endolymphatic sac surgery mentioned in the literature.

The key document questioning endolymphatic sac surgery is an article by Thomsen et al. published in 1981 [13]. In this placebo-controlled trial, no difference was found between endolymphatic sac decompression and mastoidectomy for Meniere's disease, and follow-up studies were added 3 and 9 years after the study and came to similar conclusions, that is, there was no difference between the actual endolymphatic sac decompression and the placebo surgical intervention. Whereas Pilsbury investigated these data again in 1983 [14] and found that endolymphatic sac decompression provided significantly better control of vertigo compared to a placebo procedure (mastoidectomy), Welling analyzed the original data again from the 1981 study and found statistically significant improvements in specific areas (notably vertigo, tinnitus, etc.) in the endolymphatic sac decompression group. In addition to Thomsen's (1981) study, another nonblinded, randomized study from the same group of scholars compared the results of endolymphatic sac decompression with tympanic tube placement as a placebo intervention [15]. In both trials, there was no statistically significant difference in response rates between endolymphatic sac decompression surgery and the placebo intervention, although overall symptoms improved in 70% of patients, so that symptomatic improvement was considered to be a nonspecific effect of all surgical interventions. Monsell et al. reported a study of 83 patients in 1988, in which the success rate was 75%. Paparella and Fina published in 2002 that endolymphatic capsule decompression surgery resulted in complete control of vertigo symptoms in 75% of patients and hearing preservation of 98% in 90% of patients, and the authors specifically highlighted that their surgical technique consisted of a complete mastoidectomy and extensive endolymphatic capsule decompression. Huang [16] reported an experience of decompression surgery in approximately 3000 cases, with vertigo symptom control after 2–3 years more than 90%. The rationale for endolymphatic sac decompression is that removal of the bone on the surface of the endolymphatic sac provides pressure relief and allows the endolymphatic sac to expand, thereby reducing episodic vertigo.

6.2 About Endolymphatic Duct Ligation Surgery

Saliba et al. described a novel nondestructive surgical technique for the treatment of Meniere's disease in 2015, which they performed endolymphatic truncation. They compared this technique to endolymphatic sac decompression in a prospective, nonblinded randomized trial. After endolymphatic sac decompression was completed, the endolymphatic vessels were exposed and ligated with two titanium clips. In this way, endolymphatic fluid accumulation in the inner ear is reduced, thereby balancing the imbalance between endolymphatic fluid production and absorption by blocking suspected overproduction of endolymphatic fluid in the sac. In Saliba's study, 35 patients underwent endolymphatic truncation and 22 underwent endolymphatic sac decompression only. Postoperative outcomes were assessed at 1 week, 6 months, 12 months, 18 months, and 24 months postoperatively, and the incidence of vertigo 6 months after endolymphatic duct occlusion and endolymphatic sac decompression was 3.5% and 80% respectively, and 3.5% and 66%, respectively, at 24 months, both with significant differences. Tinnitus and ear stuffiness were significantly improved in the truncated group compared to the control group at 24 months. As for the hearing results, there was no difference between the two groups. Intraoperative cerebrospinal fluid effusion occurred in 14% of the patients during dural preparation, and postoperative symptoms of posterior semicircular canal BPPV were observed in 11 out of 35 patients; no further serious complications were observed in either group. According to Saliba et al., the new method of blocking the endolymphatic vessels is clearly superior to endolymphatic sac decompression in controlling vertigo symptoms. From this literature, endolymphatic vessel occlusion appears to be an effective surgical technique, demonstrating good vertigo control and significantly improving postoperative quality of life, but its reported results in vertigo control are similar to other previous literature on the efficacy of endolymphatic sac decompression. However, its surgical technique is clearly more challenging and carries a higher risk of intraoperative cerebrospinal fluid leakage than endolymphatic sac decompression.

References

1. Rown JS. A ten year statistical follow-up of 245 consecutive cases of endolymphatic shunt and decompression with 328 consecutive cases of labyrinthectomy. Laryngoscope. 1983;93(11 Pt 1):1419–24.
2. Brinson GM, Chen DA, Arriaga MA. Endolymphatic mastoid shunt versus endolymphatic sac decompression for Ménière's disease. Otolaryngol Head Neck Surg. 2007;136(3):415–21.
3. Chung JW, Fayad J, Linthicum F, et al. Histopathology after endolymphatic sac surgery for Ménière's syndrome. Otol Neurotol. 2011;32(4):660–4.
4. Portmann G. Surgical treatment of vertigo by opening of the saccus endolymphaticus. Arch Otolaryngol. 1969;89(6):809–15.
5. Hallpike CS, Cairns H. Observations on the pathology of Ménière's syndrome. Proc R Soc Med. 1938;31(11):1317–36.
6. House WF. Subarachnoid shunt for drainage of endolymphatic hydrops. A preliminary report. Laryngoscope. 1962;72:713–29.
7. Lundquist PG, Kimura R, Wersaell J. Experiments in endolymph circulation. Acta Otolaryngol Suppl. 1964;188(s188):198.
8. Sennaroglu L, Sennaroglu G, Gursel B, et al. Intratympanic dexamethasone, intratympanic gentamicin, and endolymphatic sac surgery for intractable vertigo in Meniere's disease. Otolaryngol Head Neck Surg. 2001;125(5):537–43.
9. Silverstein H, Jackson LE. Vestibular nerve section. Otolaryngol Clin N Am. 2002;35(3):655–73.
10. Jackson CG, Dickins JR, McMenomey SO, et al. Endolymphatic system shunting: a long-term profile of the Denver Inner Ear Shunt. Am J Otolaryngol. 1996;17(1):85–8.
11. Smith DR, Pyle GM. Outcome-based assessment of endolymphatic sac surgery for Meniere's disease. Laryngoscope. 1997;107(9):1210–6.
12. Pensak ML, Friedman RA. The role of endolymphatic mastoid shunt surgery in the managed care era. Am J Otolaryngol. 1998;19(3):337–40.
13. Thomsen J, Bretlau P, Tos M, et al. Placebo effect in surgery for Ménière's disease. A double-blind, placebo-controlled study on endolymphatic sac shunt surgery. Arch Otolaryngol. 1981;107(5):271–7.
14. Thomsen J, Bretlau P, Tos M, et al. Ménière's disease: a 3-year follow-up of patients in a double-blind placebo-controlled study on endolymphatic sac shunt surgery. Adv Otorhinolaryngol. 1983;30:350–4.
15. Thomsen J, Bretlau P, Tos M, et al. Ménière's disease: endolymphatic sac decompression compared with sham (placebo) decompression. Ann N Y Acad Sci. 1981;374:820–30.
16. Huang TS. Endolymphatic sac surgery for Meniere's disease: experience with over 3000 cases. Otolaryngol Clin N Am. 2002;35(3):591–606.

7 Some Understanding of Meniere's Disease

Lin Han, Xingli Li, and Lisheng Yu

Meniere's disease is a common inner ear disorder characterized by recurrent vertigo, fluctuating hearing loss, tinnitus, and a feeling of fullness in the ear, severely impacting patients' quality of life. Diagnosis currently relies on clinical symptoms and pure-tone audiometry. Despite advancements in vestibular function and imaging tests, they are insufficient for confirming Meniere's disease. Since its initial description by Prosper Meniere in the early nineteenth century, the etiology, diagnosis, and treatment of Meniere's disease have been challenging. The discovery of its comorbidity with vestibular migraine and the high incidence of bilateral cases have shifted treatment goals from primarily controlling vertigo attacks to preserving inner ear function as much as possible. Destructive treatments like vestibular nerve section and labyrinthectomy are gradually being phased out.

L. Han · X. Li · L. Yu (✉)
Department of Otorhinolaryngology, Head and Neck Surgery, People's Hospital, Peking University, Beijing, China

7.1 In 2017, China's New Guidelines Categorized Meniere's Disease into Clinical Diagnosis and Suspected Diagnosis, Aligning with Clinical Requirements

The concept of graded diagnosis for Meniere's disease was first proposed by the American Academy of Otolaryngology-Head and Neck Surgery (AA0 HNS) in 1995, dividing it into four levels: certain, definite, probable, and possible Meniere's disease [1]. China's 2006 "Diagnostic Criteria and Therapeutic Effect Evaluation of Meniere's Disease (2006, Guiyang)" introduced clinical diagnosis and "Meniere's disease to be diagnosed [2]." The 2015 guidelines from the Barany Society categorized Meniere's disease as "clinical diagnosis of Meniere's disease" and "suspected diagnosis of Meniere's disease" [3]. The graded diagnosis of Meniere's disease aligns with clinical practice, considering differences in disease progression and clinical presentation, thereby improving diagnostic accuracy. To meet clinical and research needs, the Chinese Society of Otorhinolaryngology-Head and Neck Surgery referenced the latest Barany guidelines and tailored them to China's specific circumstances, ultimately establishing the updated "Diagnosis and Treatment Guidelines for Meniere's Disease (2017)," which also distinguish between clinical

L. Yu (ed.), *Progress in Postauricular Administration*, Experts' Perspectives on Medical Advances,
https://doi.org/10.1007/978-981-95-5102-6_7

and suspected diagnoses [4]. Eliminating previous definite diagnosis categories in the new guidelines reflects current clinical requirements, as pathological diagnosis of Meniere's disease is impractical. While endolymphatic hydrops is its pathophysiological basis, many other conditions, such as migraine, autoimmune inner ear disease, and sudden deafness, can also present with endolymphatic hydrops. Therefore, the presence of endolymphatic hydrops does not necessarily indicate Meniere's disease. Postmortem reports from abroad indicate endolymphatic hydrops in 6% of cases, whereas the incidence rate of Meniere's disease is only 0.2%.

Table 7.1 Clinical subtypes of Meniere's disease

	Clinical subtypes (unilateral)	Clinical subtypes (bilateral)
Type 1	Sporadic MD without migraines or autoimmune disease	Bilateral successive SNHL without migraines or autoimmune disease
Type 2	Late-onset MD	Bilateral synchronous SNHL without migraines or autoimmune disease
Type 3	Familial MD	Familial MD
Type 4	MD with migraines	MD with migraines
Type 5	MD with other autoimmune diseases	MD with other autoimmune diseases

7.2 The Choice of Different Frequencies Does Not Statistically Affect the Hearing Staging of Meniere's Disease But Using the Frequency Selection in the New Guidelines Is Still Recommended

Meniere's disease is a clinical syndrome characterized by recurrent vertigo, fluctuating hearing loss, and symptoms such as tinnitus and/or a sensation of fullness in the ear. Hearing loss and ear fullness symptoms may accompany vertigo attacks or occur between episodes. Vertigo attacks are typically more common in the early years of the disease, while variability in hearing loss and vestibular function is significant among different patients. The variability in these clinical symptoms complicates the staging and assessment of treatment efficacy for Meniere's disease.

In the 1995 American Academy of Otolaryngology-Head and Neck Surgery (AAO-HNS) guidelines, patients were first categorized into Stages I–IV based on pure-tone thresholds (Table 7.1). This classification system allows for assessing the disease stage based on hearing status and aids in treatment decisions. China's 2006 Guiyang standards categorized Meniere's disease into early, middle, and late stages based on changes in patient hearing characteristics. The 2015 Barany Society guidelines did not introduce disease staging. However, they emphasized the importance of assessing hearing thresholds below 2000 Hz, with stricter criteria for the degree of hearing loss compared to previous standards aimed at distinguishing vestibular migraine. The 2017 new guidelines adopted the staging criteria from the 1995 AAO-HNS guidelines, dividing patients into stages I–IV based on pure-tone thresholds. Hearing thresholds are crucial factors in selecting Meniere's disease treatment plans and assessing treatment efficacy, making staging by hearing thresholds beneficial for clinical practice. The 1995 AAO-HNS guidelines recommended evaluating hearing thresholds at four frequencies: 500 Hz, 1 kHz, 2 kHz, and 3 kHz. The new guidelines primarily recommend three frequencies, 500 Hz, 1 kHz, and 2 kHz, explaining that this decision primarily references international standards that emphasize low-frequency hearing loss and exclude 3 kHz, a frequency not routinely tested clinically, to facilitate guideline application at the grassroots level. The selection of 3 kHz is mainly because human speech frequencies primarily range from 500 to 3 kHz.

To clarify whether these different frequency selections affect staging, we analyzed Meniere's disease patients admitted to our department from 1996 to 2016 [5]. Patients were grouped based on different frequency selections into five groups: Group I included 500 Hz, 1 kHz, 2 kHz, and

3 kHz (as proposed by the 1995 AAO-HNS guidelines for the diagnosis and efficacy evaluation of Meniere's disease); Group II included 250 Hz, 500 Hz, 1 kHz, 2 kHz, and 3 kHz (from the 2006 Guiyang version of Meniere's disease diagnosis and treatment guidelines); Group III included 250 Hz, 500 Hz, 1 kHz, and 2 kHz (according to the 2015 Barany Society guidelines for Meniere's disease diagnosis); Group IV included 500 Hz, 1 kHz, 2 kHz, and 4 kHz; and Group V included 500 Hz, 1 kHz, and 2 kHz (from the 2017 Meniere's disease diagnosis and treatment guidelines). Hearing staging was calculated based on the mean values of selected frequencies, and statistical analysis revealed that the choice of different frequencies did not have a statistically significant impact on hearing staging. However, when 250 Hz was included in the staging, there was an increased likelihood of higher staging, possibly due to significant cochlear hydrops in Meniere's disease patients, resulting in more severe low-frequency hearing loss.

Hearing staging is crucial in selecting Meniere's disease treatment plans and assessing treatment efficacy. Although our study suggests that choosing different pure-tone audiometry frequencies does not significantly affect staging, we still recommend using the latest guideline frequencies, especially when 3 kHz testing is inconvenient or not feasible. Of course, facilities with the capability can still conduct 3 kHz threshold testing to accumulate clinical data further, providing a reference for future improvements in diagnostic criteria.

7.3 The Increased Incidence of Autoimmune Diseases in Patients with Meniere's Disease Supports the Potential Immunological Origins of Meniere's Disease

The pathogenesis of Meniere's disease remains unclear, with various theories, including increasing research on the role of autoimmunity and immune mechanisms in its development. In autoimmune diseases, the immune response targets the host's cells and tissues. Tomoda K proposed that the structural components of the inner ear could act as autoantigens, targets of the host's autoimmune system [6]. The immune response can involve cellular immunity, activating phagocytes and antigen-specific T lymphocytes, or humoral immunity, involving antibodies produced by B cells of the immune system. Studies by Arnold W suggest that the inner ear exhibits immune activity, with deposits of immunoglobulins and leukocytes detected in the endolymphatic sac area, surrounded by a dense network of lymphatic vessels [7]. Animal experiments by Tomiyama S demonstrate immune responses in the endolymphatic sac [8].

Previous research on Meniere's disease has identified numerous factors contributing to autoimmune diseases, including genetics, environment, hormones, and immune responses, with stress considered a triggering factor for autoimmune reactions [9]. Some large-scale epidemiological studies suggest an association between Meniere's disease and autoimmune diseases. Research by Gazquez reported an increased prevalence of systemic autoimmune diseases such as rheumatoid arthritis, systemic lupus erythematosus, and ankylosing spondylitis among Meniere's disease patients compared to the general population [10]. In 2014, Tyrrell JS surveyed a large sample of Meniere's disease patients, assessing prevalence, associated factors, and comorbidities using UK Biobank data. They found that Meniere's disease patients were more likely to report at least one allergy, autoimmune disease, or autonomic nervous system disorder. Common diseases include arthritis, chronic fatigue syndrome, mixed pollen allergies, rhinitis, eczema, drug allergies, irritable bowel syndrome, gastroesophageal reflux disease, migraine, and psoriasis. The likelihood of Meniere's disease patients developing these diseases nearly doubled [11]. Increased rates of autoimmune diseases have also been observed in familial Meniere's disease patients [12]. Multiple studies report an increased incidence of allergies among Meniere's disease patients, suggesting a possible role for IgE-mediated allergic reactions as a contributing factor [13]. Dereberg et al. reported symptom improvements in Meniere's disease following antiallergic treatments [14]. Similar to many known autoimmune diseases, Meniere's disease exhibits a fluctuating natural course, leading to the gradual progressive deterioration of affected organs. However, there are also reports of negative findings regarding the relationship between autoimmunity, allergies, and Meniere's disease [15].

Support for the autoimmune theory of Meniere's disease includes (1) increased incidence of autoimmune diseases in Meniere's disease patients, (2) elevated levels of antibodies and immune complexes in Meniere's disease patients, (3) associations between Meniere's disease and HLA typing and genetic polymorphisms [16], and (4) favorable responses to glucocorticoid treatment in some Meniere's disease patients. Nevertheless, many studies are small-scale, and there are conflicting results regarding antibodies, HLA types, and genetic polymorphisms [17]. Immunological factors likely play a role in the pathogenesis of Meniere's disease; however, further research is needed to determine the extent and mechanisms of autoimmune involvement in the onset of Meniere's disease.

7.4 Multiple Genes Are Known to Be Involved in familial Meniere's Disease, While the Relationship Between Sporadic Meniere's Disease and Genetic Factors Requires Further Investigation

Meniere's disease exhibits significant familial clustering. Paparella's study of 500 Meniere's disease patients found a familial tendency in 20% of cases. Although genetics play a role in the pathogenesis of this disease, the inheritance patterns are diverse. Several studies support that genetic factors contribute to phenotypic variation [17, 18]. Up to 10% of patients may have confirmed familial aggregation involving first- and second-degree relatives [19]. Most of these pedigrees exhibit an autosomal dominant inheritance pattern with incomplete penetrance and variability [20]. The genetics of Meniere's disease are complex, and extensive research has been conducted on both familial and sporadic cases to elucidate the molecular basis of the disease.

Meniere's disease is primarily sporadic, yet approximately 9–10% of cases in European populations are familial [21]. Distinguishing clinical features between familial and sporadic cases is challenging. Several allelic variations in innate immune response genes MICA, TLR10, and NFKB1 affect the auditory outcomes of sporadic Meniere's disease [22–24]. The channelopathy hypothesis supports aquaporins (AQPs) as molecular targets in Meniere's disease. AQPs facilitate water and solute transport along osmotic gradients, with four types (AQP1–AQP4) expressed in the human inner ear. Vasopressin regulates AQP water permeability, and it has been reported that vasopressin increases before vertiginous attacks in Meniere's disease. Vertiginous attacks may result from interactions between increased vasopressin release and allelic variations in AQP genes [25, 26]. A case-control study identified susceptibility to Meniere's disease associated with a common variant of the Add1 gene, which encodes a cytoskeletal protein interacting with the Na+-K+-ATPase transporter, thereby affecting transport activity. However, these findings have not been consistently replicated in independent cohort studies, underscoring the heterogeneity of genetic factors [27].

Familial Meniere's disease (FMD) should be considered when at least two family members (first or second degree) meet all defined or possible Meniere's disease criteria. Most FMD pedigrees exhibit an autosomal dominant inheritance pattern, with some families also showing mitochondrial and autosomal recessive inheritance patterns [28]. Linkage studies of FMD identified candidate loci at 5q14–5q15 in a German family and 12p12.3 in a Swedish family [29]. Requena et al. identified mutations in the DTNA and FAM136A genes through exome sequencing in a Spanish family with autosomal dominant inheritance [30]. DTNA encodes a protein involved in interactions with transmembrane proteins and actin filaments in the basolateral membrane of epithelial cells, which is related to tight junction remodeling. FAM136A is a mitochondria-associated protein with an unknown function. FAM136A and DTNA proteins are expressed in the ampulla of the rat semicircular canal. Further research is needed to elucidate the roles of DTNA and FAM136A genes in sporadic Meniere's disease patients. Currently, six genes (COCH, DPT, DTNA, FAM136A, PRKCB, and SEMA3D) have been identified as associated with familial Meniere's disease through exome sequencing and bioinformatics tools [19–21].

Genetic factors play a significant role in the pathogenesis of familial Meniere's disease, supported by confirmation of multiple genes through exome sequencing. The role of genetic factors in sporadic Meniere's disease remains heterogeneous and requires further investigation.

7.5 Meniere's Disease Is a Heterogeneous Disorder That Can Be Classified into Different Clinical Subtypes Based on Distinct Clinical Features, Which May Benefit Future Treatments and Clinical Research

Meniere's disease often coexists with various comorbidities such as migraines or autoimmune diseases (AD) [31]. Epidemiological associations between Meniere's disease and migraines, as well as several autoimmune diseases, support the hypothesis of expanded phenotypes in Meniere's disease [32]. It suggests that symptoms of Meniere's disease extend beyond auditory-vestibular aspects, as initially reported by Meniere in female cases presenting with headaches. Using cluster analysis, Frejo defined clinical subtypes of unilateral and bilateral Meniere's disease patients. Based on clinical predictors such as delayed-onset Meniere's disease, family history of Meniere's disease, history of migraines, and autoimmune diseases, five potential pathogenetically significant subtypes were identified for unilateral Meniere's disease patients, as well as five subtypes for bilateral Meniere's disease patients (Figs. 7.1 and 7.2). These observed clinical variations confirm previous epidemiological studies and indicate that genetics and autoimmune factors independently promote the development of Meniere's disease.

7.5.1 Clinical Subtypes of Unilateral Meniere's Disease

(1) UMD 1 type is most common and includes sporadic Meniere's disease patients without a history of migraines or autoimmune diseases and no family history. Further research is needed on this large subgroup of sporadic cases to determine their pathogenic factors.

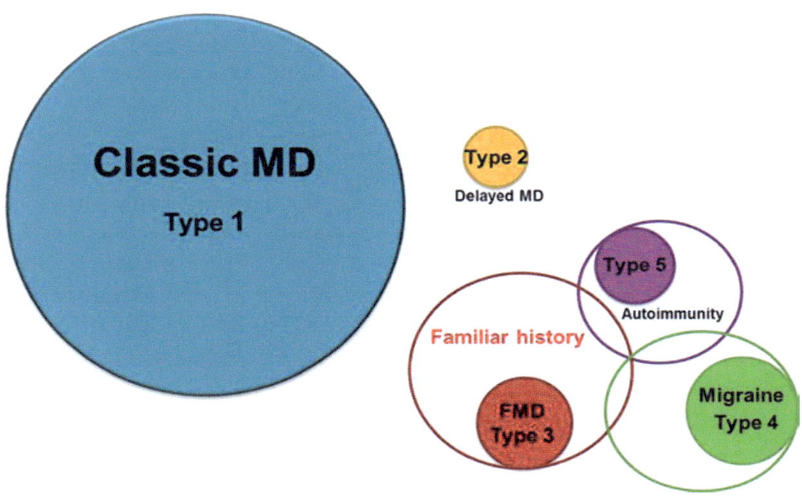

Fig. 7.1 Subtypes of unilateral Meniere's disease

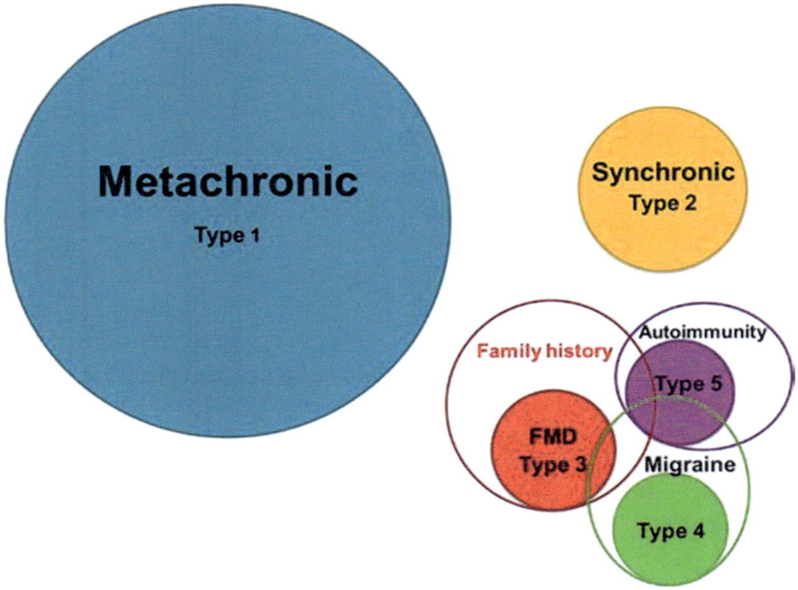

Fig. 7.2 Subtypes of bilateral Meniere's disease

(2) UMD 2 type: Late-onset Meniere's disease (previously termed delayed endolymphatic hydrops), relatively rare. Mostly sporadic Meniere's disease with no history of migraines. Autoimmune diseases are observed in only 10% of patients, similar to the general population.

(3) UMD 3 type includes all familial Meniere's disease patients. Average hearing thresholds at diagnosis are around 30 dB HL, suggesting mild fluctuating hearing loss in these patients. This type can be divided into two subtypes: UMD3a type without migraines, accounting for 78%, and UMD3b type with migraines, accounting for 22%. Familial Meniere's disease often exhibits autosomal dominant inheritance with incomplete penetrance.

(4) UMD 4 type: Sporadic Meniere's disease with comorbid migraines. Forty-one percent of UMD 4 type patients have autoimmune diseases. Managing these patients who have sporadic Meniere's disease combined with migraines and autoimmune diseases presents challenges. This vestibular migraine comorbidity group may share common pathophysiological mechanisms. Meniere's disease patients may exhibit migraine symptoms even during vertiginous attacks, which complicates the differential diagnosis between vestibular migraine and Meniere's disease [33].

(5) UMD 5 type: Considered autoimmune Meniere's disease, all patients have one or more concurrent autoimmune diseases, and all are sporadic cases without migraines.

This classification system still has limitations. Some patients cannot be classified into any group and are thus excluded from the model. The largest group (UMD 1 type) lacks distinctive features associated with any specific clinical characteristics or etiologies. Lastly, there is a 10% overlap between UMD 3 type and UMD 5 type cases (familial Meniere's disease with autoimmune diseases but without migraines).

7.5.2 Clinical Subtypes of Bilateral Meniere's Disease

Frejo L proposed a new classification of bilateral Meniere's disease (BMD) into five groups with potential pathogenic significance, which may improve the diagnostic process and management of bilateral Meniere's disease patients:

(1) BMD1 type (asynchronous SNHL): Most common clinically. Sporadic Meniere's disease patients without a family history, migraines, or autoimmune disease history, experiencing successive hearing loss in both ears. The average age of onset is 46 years, significantly higher than type 3, 4, or 5.
(2) BMD2 type (synchronous SNHL): Sporadic Meniere's disease patients with synchronous hearing loss in both ears, without migraines or autoimmune disease history. They exhibit fluctuating bilateral hearing loss resembling autoimmune inner ear disease. BMD2-type patients show vascular risk features, with 50% having hypertension and 53% having dyslipidemia.
(3) BMD3 type (familial Meniere's disease) includes all patients with a family history of Meniere's disease, subdivided based on the presence of migraines into two subgroups (3a Meniere's disease with migraines, 82%, 3b Meniere's disease without migraines, 18%).
(4) BMD4 type (Meniere's disease with migraines): Associated with migraines in all cases but without a family history of Meniere's disease. This group may overlap with vestibular migraine (VM) and may share common pathophysiological mechanisms.
(5) BMD5 type (Meniere's disease with AD) includes all patients with autoimmune comorbidities, of which 71% are sporadic and 29% have familial Meniere's disease.

Identifying different subgroups of UMD or BMD patients is the first step in improving patient selection for genetic and immunological research and improving randomized clinical trials (RCTs). Further phenotype analysis of these clinical variations is needed better to understand the clinical heterogeneity of Meniere's disease. Notably, the sporadic BMD1 type, which constitutes the majority of MD patients, is a focus of future research, whether in terms of etiology, treatment, or other aspects, and requires further investigation.

7.5.3 Classification Based on Peripheral Blood Cytokines

Different subtypes of Meniere's disease (MD) patients exhibit varying immune system function or response levels. It has been suggested that hypersensitivity reactions also play a role in the pathogenesis of MD. In a 2000 epidemiological study by Dereberg, 58% of MD patients had a history of allergies, and 41% showed positive skin prick test results. The study found associations between MD and inhalant allergens as well as food allergens [34, 35]. Topuz discovered that skin prick tests could induce auditory symptoms such as tinnitus or ear fullness in 62% of MD patients, with 77% of patients exhibiting elevated endolymphatic pressure measured by cochlear hydrops [36]. Keles et al. also assessed the role of hypersensitivity reactions in the pathogenesis of MD. They found significant differences in lymphocyte subsets (CD4, CD4/CD8, CD23), IFN-γ, and IL-4 levels in MD patients compared to controls [37]. Fuse analyzed intracellular cytokine levels in acute low-frequency hearing loss (ALHL) and MD patients, revealing an imbalance in Th1/Th2 responses in ALHL patients and increased NK cell activity in MD patients [38].

In 2017, Frejo et al. studied the effects of allergen extracts (*Aspergillus* and *Penicillium*) on cytokine release and gene expression profiles in MD patients [39]. They found that baseline levels of IL-1β, IL-1RA, IL-6, and TNF-α were higher in MD patients compared to healthy controls, and IL-1β levels showed a bimodal distribution suggesting two distinct subgroups (high IL-1β vs. low IL-1β). Both fungal extracts significantly stimulated TNF-α release in MD patients, and based on IL-1β baseline levels, different gene expression profiles were observed in peripheral blood mononuclear cells of MD patients. Elevated baseline levels of specific proinflammatory cytokines in MD patients may trigger additional TNF-α release, inducing or exacerbating inflammation in the endolymphatic sac or vestibular ligaments, leading to endolymphatic hydrops. Frejo's earlier research identified five clinical subtypes, with unilateral MD type 1 being the most common clinical variant, and most patients with elevated IL-1β belonged to MD type 1 (83.4%). The immune system function or immune response levels differ among different subtypes of Meniere's disease patients, and autoimmune reactions in the inner ear may be a pathophysiological basis for the high IL-1β subtype.

Classifying based on inflammatory factors also supports the argument that MD is a heterogeneous disease. Differences in levels of proinflammatory cytokines and immune responses to specific pathogens (including fungi) may explain why some patients respond effectively to antihistamines like betahistine while others do not. Furthermore, patients treated with immunotherapy experience improved duration and frequency of vertigo attacks. Therefore, evaluating allergic responses in MD patients and incorporating the use of antihistamines or immunotherapy into treatment plans aimed at controlling vertigo attacks should be considered.

7.6 Inner Ear MRI Gadolinium Enhancement Can Objectively Determine the Presence of Endolymphatic Hydrops But Cannot Serve as the Definitive Objective Criterion and Basis for Diagnosing Meniere's Disease (MD)

Radiological examinations such as CT scans can exclude congenital inner ear malformations and tumors and assess pneumatization of the mastoid, also revealing the condition of the endolymphatic duct and perilymphatic spaces; poor pneumatization may suggest underdeveloped endolymphatic ducts. Routine inner ear MRI scans can rule out vestibular schwannoma or endolymphatic sac tumors, among other diseases [40].

Administering gadolinium contrast agent followed by inner ear MRI enables objective assessment of endolymphatic hydrops, marking a significant advancement in MD diagnostics in recent years. Studies have confirmed the effectiveness of this technique in defining endolymphatic hydrops [41, 42]. Initial administration involves intravenous injection of gadolinium-based contrast agents (GBCAs) followed by enhanced MRI; administering double-dose gadolinium requires a 4-h delay. Advantages include the ability to assess both ears, yet high doses of gadolinium pose systemic toxicity risks, and post-injection image quality of GBCAs may be unsatisfactory. In 2007, Nakashima et al. suggested evaluating the inner ear with 3T magnetic resonance imaging (MRI) after intratympanic gadolinium injection; gadolinium entering through the round window membrane distinguishes boundaries between endolymph and perilymph. While T2-weighted images represent perilymph and endolymph, bright signals on 3D-FLAIR images represent perilymph, with dark signals inside indicating endolymph. When endolymphatic expansion exceeds 33%, endolymphatic hydrop is diagnosed. Traditional intratympanic GBCA injections occasionally result in uptake failure. In 2019, Jing Zou et al. obtained high-quality endolymphatic hydrop images within 8 min after administering a 0.1 ml, 20-fold diluted gadolinium diethylenetriamine pentaacetic acid (Gd-DTPA) via the tympanic membrane puncture and irrigation catheter into the upper part of the inner ear [43].

However, the clinical application still faces several issues: (1) This technique provides semi-quantitative evaluation, subject to subjective factors in distinguishing hydrop and nonhydrop images, with no unified standard and method for judging endolymphatic hydrops; (2) negative results may occur due to short disease course or early-stage mild MD. Gadolinium enhancement best visualizes the cochlear basal turn and vestibule, but it displays the superior turn poorly. Early MD is primarily low-frequency hearing loss (cochlear apex hydrops, as it has a cochlear mouth, so it is easier to hernia here. This is the main reason for early MD to show low-frequency hearing loss). Therefore, inner ear gadolinium enhancement is not sensitive to early

MD. Positive rates of more than three periods are high. Apart from the most critical problem, the presence of endolymphatic hydrops is not a diagnostic of Meniere's disease. It can also be seen in perioral migraine and low-frequency sensorineural hearing loss patients, as well as in healthy subjects. Therefore, endolymphatic hydrops are not a specific manifestation of Meniere's disease. An asymptomatic MRI found that endolymphatic hydrops cannot diagnose Meniere's disease. Therefore, while the technology can relatively objectively determine the presence of endolymphatic hydrops, it is a good auxiliary diagnostic technology. However, the diagnosis of Meniere's disease mainly relies on medical history and hearing tests, as highlighted in the 2015 Meniere's disease diagnostic criteria and China's new diagnostic criteria in 2017. Therefore, this examination clearly cannot be an objective criterion and basis for diagnosing Meniere's disease.

7.7 Meniere's Disease and Vestibular Migraine Are Two Common Vestibular Disorders in Otolaryngology

In this chapter, we have previously compared the characteristics of these two diseases. Both are diagnosed symptomatically and share similarities in etiology, triggers, and clinical manifestations, making their differentiation particularly challenging, especially in the early stages of the disease.

The critical difference lies in the fact that Meniere's disease causes irreversible deterioration of inner ear function, whereas vestibular migraine generally does not result in permanent inner ear functional decline, being considered a functional disorder. Vestibular migraine presents with transient vestibular dysfunction and symptoms overlapping with Meniere's disease during attacks. Additionally, migraine, episodic vertigo, and Meniere's disease (including in monozygotic twins) often cluster within families, supporting a genetic predisposition to both disorders [44]. Epidemiological studies report that approximately 56% of Meniere's disease patients experience migraine; familial susceptibility is presumed in both conditions. Migraine itself can cause episodic vertigo, with a prevalence of vestibular migraine estimated at 1% of the general population. The coexistence of these two diseases in clinical practice is not uncommon [45]. Many Meniere's disease patients experience headaches, with or without migraine-like characteristics of vertigo attacks, leading some to consider these conditions as clinical features of the same disease process. Literature reports a high prevalence of migraine in Meniere's disease [46, 47]. Furthermore, cases of Meniere's disease with concurrent vestibular migraine have been described, suggesting common pathophysiological mechanisms between the two. It has been reported that migraine may also present with mild inner ear hydrops. Psychological factors such as stress or anxiety are believed to trigger vertigo attacks [48, 49].

In our department, among 103 confirmed Meniere's disease patients who underwent hospitalization surgery due to frequent vertigo attacks, the distribution was as follows: 48 cases (46.6%) with Meniere's disease combined with vestibular migraine, 18 cases (17.5%) with likely vestibular migraine, and 37 cases (35.9%) with isolated Meniere's disease. Among patients with Meniere's disease combined with vestibular migraine, the frequency of vertigo attacks was 7.1 times per month (distinguished from patients with isolated Meniere's disease and those with likely vestibular migraine). Patients with Meniere's disease combined with vestibular migraine all had a history of migraine attacks with or without hearing loss: 41 cases of unilateral headache, 45 cases of throbbing headache, and 12 cases of visual aura. The incidence of vestibular migraine in female Meniere's disease patients was 7.92 times higher than in male Meniere's disease patients [50].

7.8 The Current Treatment Options for Meniere's Disease Can Be Divided into Sequential Protocol-Based Selection and Selection Based on the Hearing Stage

The treatment of Meniere's disease is still under exploration. Lifestyle changes, systemic drug therapy, conservative surgical treatment, and other noninvasive treatments can improve vertigo for most patients [51, 52]. The treatment guidelines for Meniere's disease published in *The Lancet* in 2008 suggest a sequential protocol-based approach, where if the effectiveness of the previous treatment plan is poor after 3 months, the following plan should be considered. According to the 1995 American Academy of Otolaryngology-Head and Neck Surgery (AAO-HNS) standards, Meniere's disease is classified into different grades based on the degree of hearing loss. Hearing staging can indicate the severity of cochlear lesions or the stage of lesion progression. In 2017, the Chinese Medical Association released the Diagnosis and Treatment Guidelines for Meniere's Disease, proposing that treatment options can be selected based on different stages of hearing loss, as shown in Table 7.2. Surgical treatment is generally considered after Stage III, with a preference for conservative surgeries such as endolymphatic sac surgery. Surgery may also be considered for Stage II patients with very frequent attacks who express a desire for surgery. A notable change in Chinese guidelines is not only focusing on controlling vertigo but also emphasizing preserving or reconstructing inner ear function (including cochlear implantation and vestibular implantation). Therefore, destructive treatments such as labyrinthectomy and vestibular nerve section should be avoided as much as possible. In 2018, the International Consensus on Meniere's Disease Treatment (ICON) in Europe classified evidence into levels (1–5) and divided treatment into five steps: Step 1, drug therapy; Step 2, intratympanic steroid therapy; Step 3, conservative surgical treatment; Step 4, destructive treatment with intratympanic gentamicin; and Step 5, destructive surgical treatment. After Step 3, treatment selection is based on the effectiveness of hearing (Fig. 7.3). The 2020 AAO-HNS Clinical Practice Guidelines for Meniere's Disease aim to improve the quality and effectiveness of MD diagnosis and treatment by using the best available clinical evidence to enhance diagnostic accuracy and select appropriate medical and surgical interventions while reducing unnecessary tests and imaging studies. Treatment selection is also carried out according to a protocol-based approach, although some commonly used treatments, such as low-pressure pulse therapy, are not recommended in the guidelines.

The goal of treating patients with Meniere's disease is to reduce the frequency and severity of vertigo attacks while minimizing hearing damage. Treatment should be tailored to the patient's symptoms and related complaints. Conservative treatment should be the first-line choice.

Table 7.2 Treatment options for Meniere's disease

Clinical staging	Treatment options
Stage I	Patient education, lifestyle improving, betahistine, diuretics, intratympanic injection of glucocorticoid, and vestibular rehabilitation training
Stage II	Patient education, lifestyle improving, betahistine, diuretics, intratympanic injection of glucocorticoid, low-pressure pulse therapy, and vestibular rehabilitation training
Stage III	Patient education, lifestyle improving, betahistine, diuretics, intratympanic injection of glucocorticoid, low-pressure pulse therapy, endolymphatic sac surgery, intratympanic injection of gentamicin, and vestibular rehabilitation training
Stage IV	Patient education, lifestyle improving, betahistine, diuretics, intratympanic injection of glucocorticoid, low-pressure pulse therapy, intratympanic injection of gentamicin, three semicircular canal occlusion, vestibular neurotomy, labyrinthectomy, and vestibular rehabilitation training

Note: Endolymphatic sac surgery can also be considered for some patients with frequent and severe vertigo attacks and a strong desire for surgery. For some frequent and severe vertigo attacks, endolymphatic sac surgery is invalid; the speech recognition rate is less than 50%; Stage III urged surgery patients can also consider three semicircular canal occlusions

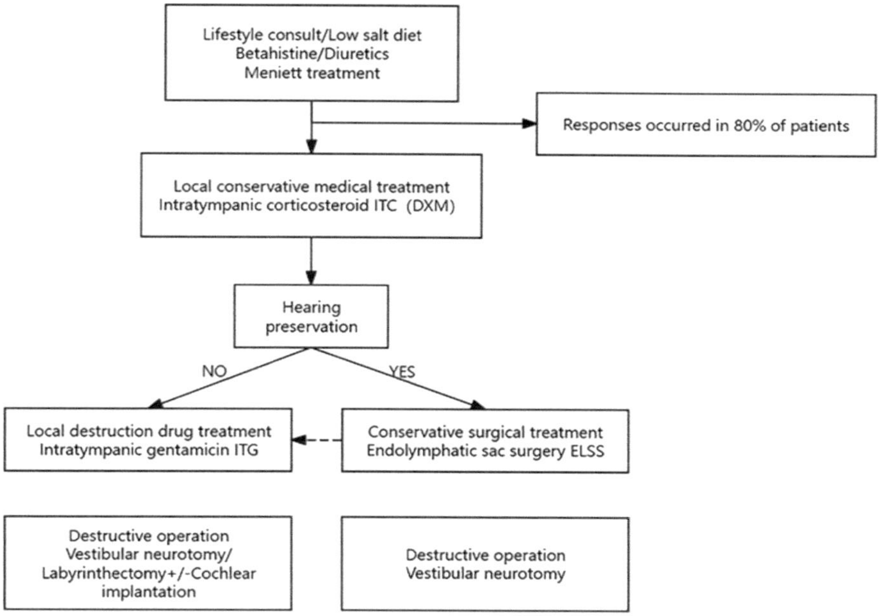

Fig. 7.3 ICON stepwise treatment

7.9 It Is Recommended to Combine Antimigraine Therapy for Meniere's Patients with Concurrent Migraines

In existing treatment guidelines and protocols for Meniere's disease, antimigraine therapy has not yet been included in the recommended drug treatment regimens. However, as mentioned earlier, literature reports that many Meniere's disease patients experience headaches with or without accompanying vertigo symptoms. A subset of Meniere's disease patients also experience vestibular migraine concurrently, with 21% of VM patients with auditory symptoms showing membranous labyrinth hydrops, suggesting a potential common pathophysiological mechanism between the two conditions. According to the clinical classification proposed by Frejo, bilateral Meniere's disease Type 3 primarily includes familial Meniere's disease, with 82% of cases being the subtype with accompanying migraines; Type 4 involves Meniere's disease with migraines and is considered to possibly overlap with VM. Currently, patients meeting diagnostic criteria for both Meniere's disease and vestibular migraine are initially diagnosed with Meniere's disease for stepwise or sequential treatment. However, considering that migraine mechanisms may be a contributing factor in the onset of Meniere's disease, combined antimigraine therapy is recommended for Meniere's patients with concurrent migraines.

7.10 When Using H1-Antihistamines to Treat Meniere's Disease, Increasing the Dosage Appropriately Is Feasible

The mechanism of preventing continued vertigo attacks with β-histamines (H1-antihistamines, most commonly betahistine) involves their H1 potentiating effect and H3 antagonistic action. The drug's action is based on its antihistaminic and vasodilatory effects in the inner ear, particularly the cochlear vascular plexus, with reports suggesting its effects on vestibular central neurons and its association with differences in proinflammatory factors and immune responses [53]. Some literature reports that β-histamines can reduce the frequency and severity of Meniere's disease attacks, while others question its effectiveness [53, 54]. Systematic reviews and meta-analyses of betahistine treatment for Meniere's disease support its ability to alleviate vertigo symptoms. Although systematic analyses indicate that many studies do not meet high-quality research standards, most studies support the effectiveness of betahistine in alleviating Meniere's disease vertigo symptoms. In a multicenter, long-term double-blind randomized controlled study by Adrion in 2016, betahistine was found to have limited control over vertigo, whether at low doses (2 * 24 mg per day) or high doses (3 * 48 mg per day). However, due to its high tolerability, low risk, and potential for promoting vestibular compensation, it continues to be widely used by many physicians and patients. The study design in this literature has significant flaws, as it selected cases of "Meniere's disease" patients with fewer than five attacks per month. Research from our department indicates that "pure" Meniere's disease does not exceed two attacks per month. Thus, when reading literature, attention should not only be paid to study results but also to study design and original data. Betahistine is popular in France, Europe, and Japan and used by many doctors in Australia, but its use is rare in the United States due to a lack of FDA approval. Betahistine is used at different doses in various centers, with literature suggesting better efficacy at a minimum dose of 48 mg/day. For severe Meniere's disease patients with inadequate response to low doses, betahistine dosage may be increased to 288–480 mg/day. Although adverse reactions to high-dose medications are rare, and some reports suggest better efficacy, these doses are not recommended for safety reasons [55]. β-Histamines can be used long-term (8–16 mg TID). Based on our experience, increasing the dosage may be considered for individual patients with poor response (informing patients about postprandial administration and contraindications such as bronchial asthma and gastric ulcer), generally achieving good therapeutic effects with doses up to 24 mg TID.

7.11 The Treatment Choice for Bilateral Meniere's Disease Should Primarily Focus on Conservative Management

Meniere's disease patients exhibit phenotypic heterogeneity, making it difficult to clearly understand the disease's onset, progression, and outcome early on. Generally, during the early stages of the disease (within 3–5 years of onset), vertigo attacks are more frequent, and balance issues may arise as the disease progresses, especially if bilateral vestibular function declines, potentially exacerbating balance impairments [56]. Most patients initially present with unilateral involvement, with contralateral ear involvement occurring several years later; however, a significant number of individuals also present with bilateral disease simultaneously [57]. Bilateral involvement is a major concern for patients due to the impact of vestibular function loss on their quality of life [58].

The reported proportion of bilateral Meniere's disease varies widely, ranging from 2% to 78%. Such discrepancies may be attributed to several factors. Firstly, there is no uniform diagnostic criterion; Paparella reported that 78% of Meniere's disease patients experience bilateral hearing loss, but clinically, only 32% meet the criteria for bilateral Meniere's disease. Another reason is the lack of standardized follow-up intervals, leading to significant variations in the natural course of the disease and the condition of patients at the time of consultation [59]. Some scholars suggest that the likelihood of developing bilateral Meniere's disease within 5 years after unilateral onset is not high, although others believe that the probability of bilateral onset increases over time [60]. Studies describe bilateral onset rates ranging from 10% to 35% within 5 years and frequencies from 20% to 46% over follow-ups of 10 years or longer. Rates of bilateral occurrence rise to 47% after over 20 years of follow-up. While the proportion of individuals affected bilaterally varies widely, most studies emphasize an increase in contralateral ear involvement with disease progression.

Previous research has often lacked sufficient numbers of bilateral patients to evaluate clinical differences between unilateral and bilateral Meniere's disease. Gazquez assessed 611 MD patients (403 unilateral, 208 bilateral) and found differences in the years of vertigo attacks between unilateral and bilateral MD patients, with median ages of reaching Stage IV being 27 years and 24 years, respectively [61]. Among patients with bilateral hearing loss, vertigo attacks persisted for more than 2 years, indicating possible involvement of both ears in disease onset. The median duration of vertigo in unilateral patients was 10 years (95% confidence interval, 8.56–11.44), significantly longer in bilateral patients (12 years (10.4–13.6)). The time course of vertigo attacks differs between unilateral and bilateral Meniere's patients, suggesting potentially longer durations of vertigo in bilateral patients.

The challenge with bilateral Meniere's disease lies in many patients initially presenting unilaterally, with delayed involvement of the contralateral ear, impacting the selection of treatment strategies. Bilateral onset occurs years later and necessitates avoiding bilateral vestibular nerve section or destructive therapies. Bilateral vestibular function decline significantly affects patient quality of life. Patients should be informed about the higher likelihood of bilateral onset when unilateral onset is initially treated. First-line treatment should prioritize conservative management, with increasing teams shifting from intratympanic gentamicin injections to steroid injections. Surgical treatment for bilateral Meniere's disease recommends initially selecting the ear with better hearing for endolymphatic sac decompression surgery to preserve inner ear function on that side before addressing the contralateral ear.

7.12 A More Accurate Evaluation of the Effectiveness of Postoperative Vertigo Control in Meniere's Disease Should Exclude Dizziness or Vertigo Caused by Other Diseases

The assessment of surgical efficacy for Meniere's disease has many shortcomings. It primarily relies on the frequency of vertigo attacks before and after treatment: comparing the number of attacks during the 18–24 months after treatment with those in the 6 months before treatment, scored accordingly. Score = (number of attacks during 18–24 months after treatment/number of attacks in the 6 months before treatment) × 100. Based on the score, the degree of vertigo control is categorized into five levels: Grade A, 0 points (complete control); Grade B, 1–40 points (basic control); Grade C, 41–80 points (partial control); Grade D, 81–120 points (uncontrolled); and Grade E, >120 points (worsening).

Therefore, for a more accurate assessment of efficacy, it is necessary to more accurately determine the number of vertigo occurrences caused by Meniere's disease before and after surgery. Currently, we know that Meniere's disease often coexists with common comorbidities such as allergies, autoimmune diseases, benign paroxysmal positional vertigo (BPPV), and migraine [62]. According to our previous studies, among 103 patients with Meniere's disease, 48 were diagnosed with vestibular migraine, with an incidence rate of 46.6%. Pyykko et al. suggest that Meniere's disease and vestibular migraine may share similar pathophysiological mechanisms. Meniere's disease and vestibular migraine are closely related, and vertigo attacks in Meniere's disease often coincide with vertigo caused by vestibular migraine. Similarly, BPPV may also be related to Meniere's disease, with a reported incidence rate as high as 26.4% among patients [63].

Therefore, to assess vertigo control, it is important to exclude vertigo caused by vestibular migraine and BPPV as much as possible. According to the latest diagnostic criteria, the duration of vertigo attacks in Meniere's disease ranges from 20 min to 12 h. Considering the duration of vertigo attacks can help exclude some types of vertigo. A study evaluated the postoperative efficacy in 121 Meniere's disease patients who underwent endolymphatic sac decompression surgery. Method 1 included all durations of vertigo attacks, while Method 2 only included attacks lasting from 20 min to 12 h. The results indicated that the effectiveness in Grades A + B was 84% in Method 2 compared to 77% in Method 1, with 64% of Grade A patients based on Method 2, significantly higher than the 36%

based on Method 1. Therefore, previous assessments may have underestimated the efficacy of endolymphatic sac surgery, especially for Grade A patients.

Excluding other types of vertigo by considering the duration of vertigo attacks is a straightforward method to obtain a more reliable assessment of efficacy. However, it should be noted that vertigo attacks from vestibular migraine may also fall within the 20-min to 12-h range, and this method does not entirely exclude vertigo caused by vestibular migraine. Compared to Meniere's disease, patients with vestibular migraine have a significantly younger age of onset, less tinnitus, ear fullness, and hearing loss but more vomiting, headaches, aura, and photophobia. Therefore, for a more accurate evaluation, factors such as hearing, triggers, and accompanying symptoms should also be included in the assessment, necessitating further research to improve methods.

Surgery often selects patients with recent and frequent attacks, while conservative treatment encompasses all types, making direct comparisons difficult. Therefore, it is recommended that future studies select patients with frequent attacks in the past 6 months and compare them after a six-month follow-up observation period, which may be more reasonable.

References

1. Committee on Hearing and Equilibrium guidelines for the diagnosis and evaluation of therapy in Meniere's disease. Otolaryngol Head Neck Surg. 1995;113(3):181–5.
2. Otolaryngology Society of Chinese Medical Association, Diagnostic basis and curative effect evaluation of Meniere disease (2006, Guiyang). Chin J Otolaryngol Head Neck Surg. 2007;42(3):163.
3. Lopez-Escamez JA, Carey J, et al. Diagnostic criteria of Meniere's disease. J Vestib Res. 2015;25:1–7.
4. Chinese Society of Otolaryngology, Guidelines for Diagnosis and Treatment of Meniere Disease (2017). Chin J Otolaryngol Head Neck Surg. 2017;52(3):167–72.
5. Han Lin, Li Xueshi, et al. Analysis of the relationship between audiological stages and selected frequencies in patients with Meniere disease. Clin Otolaryngol Head Neck Surg.
6. Tomoda K, Suzuka Y, Iwai H, et al. Meniere's disease and autoimmunity: clinical study and survey. Acta Otolaryngol Suppl. 1993;500:31–4.
7. Tomiyama S, Harris JP. The endolymphatic sac: its importance in inner ear immune responses. Laryngoscope. 1986;96(June (6)):685–91.
8. Arnold W, Pfaltz R, Altermatt HJ. Evidence of serum antibodies against inner ear tissues in the blood of patients with certain sensorineural hearing disorders. Acta Otolaryngol. 1985;99(March–April (3–4)):437–44.
9. Stojanovich L, Marisavljevich D. Stress as a trigger of autoimmune disease. Autoimmun Rev. 2008;7(January (3)):209–13.
10. Gazquez I, Soto-Varela A, Aran I, et al. High prevalence of systemic autoimmune diseases in patients with Meniere's disease. PLoS One. 2011;6(10):e26759.
11. Tyrrell JS, Whinney DJ, Ukoumunne OC, et al. Prevalence, associated factors, and comorbid conditions for Meniere's disease. Ear Hear. 2014;35(July–August (4)):e162–9.
12. Hietikko E, Sorri M, Mannikko M, et al. Higher prevalence of autoimmune diseases and longer spells of vertigo in patients affected with familial Meniere's disease: a clinical comparison of familial and sporadic Meniere's disease. Am J Audiol. 2014;23(June (2)):232–7.
13. Duke W. Meniere's syndrome caused by allergy. JAMA. 1923;81:2179–82.
14. Derebery MJ, Berliner KI. Prevalence of allergy in Meniere's disease. Otolaryngol Head Neck Surg. 2000;123(July (1 Pt. 1)):69–75.
15. Ruckenstein MJ. Immunologic aspects of Meniere's disease. Am J Otolaryngol. 1999;20(May–June (3)):161–5.
16. Flook M, Lopez-Escamez JA. Meniere's disease: Genetics and the immune system. Curr Otorhinolaryngol Rep. 2018;6:24.
17. Boulassel MR, Alost M, Tomasi JP, et al. No increased serum levels of antifood antibodies in patients with Meniere's disease. ORL J Otorhinolaryngol Relat Spec. 2001;63(January–February (1)):19–24.
18. Gallego-Martinez A, Espinosa-Sanchez JM, Lopez-Escamez JA. Genetic contribution to vestibular diseases. J Neurol. 2018. https://doi.org/10.1007/s00415-018-8842-7. [Epub ahead of print].
19. Martín-Sierra C, Requena T, Frejo L, et al. A novel missense variant in PRKCB segregates low-frequency hearing loss in an autosomal dominant family with Meniere's disease. Hum Mol Genet. 2016;25:3407–15.
20. Martín-Sierra C, Gallego-Martinez A, Requena T, et al. Variable expressivity and genetic heterogeneity involving DPT and SEMA3D genes in autosomal dominant familial Meniere's disease. Eur J Hum Genet. 2017;25:200–7.
21. Requena T, Espinosa-Sanchez JM, Cabrera S, et al. Familial clustering and genetic heterogeneity in Meniere's disease. Clin Genet. 2014;85(3):245–52.

22. Gazquez I, Moreno A, Aran I, et al. MICA-STR A.4 is associated with slower hearing loss progression in patients with Meniere's disease. Otol Neurotol Off Publ Am Otol Soc Am Neurotol Soc Eur Acad Otol Neurotol. 2012;33(2):223–9.
23. Requena T, Gazquez I, Moreno A, et al. Allelic variants in TLR10 gene may influence bilateral affectation and clinical course of Meniere's disease. Immunogenetics. 2013;65(5):345–55.
24. Cabrera S, Sanchez E, Requena T, et al. Intronic variants in the NFKB1 gene may influence hearing forecast in patients with unilateral sensorineural hearing loss in Meniere's disease. PLoS One. 2014;9(11):e112171.
25. Knepper MA, Inoue T. Regulation of aquaporin-2 water channel trafficking by vasopressin. Curr Opin Cell Biol. 1997;9(4):560–4.
26. Takeda T, Takeda S, Kakigi A, et al. Hormonal aspects of Meniere's disease on the basis of clinical and experimental studies. ORL J Oto Rhino Laryngol Relat Spec. 2010;71(Suppl 1):1–9.
27. Teggi R, Lanzani C, Zagato L, et al. Gly460Trp alpha-adducin mutation as a possible mechanism leading to endolymphatic hydrops in Meniere's syndrome. Otol Neurotol Off Publ Am Otol Soc Am Neurotol Soc Eur Acad Otol Neurotol. 2008;29(6):824–8.
28. Arweiler-Harbeck D, Horsthemke B, Jahnke K, et al. Genetic aspects of familial Meniere's disease. Otol Neurotol Off Publ Am Otol Soc Am Neurotol Soc Eur Acad Otol Neurotol. 2011;32(4):695–700.
29. Klar J, Frykholm C, Friberg U, et al. A Meniere's disease gene linked to chromosome 12p12.3. Am J Med Genet Part B Neuropsychiatr Genet Off Publ Int Soc Psychiatr Genet. 2006;141B(5):463–7.
30. Requena T, Cabrera S, Martin-Sierra C, et al. Identification of two novel mutations in FAM136A and DTNA genes in autosomal-dominant familial Meniere's disease. Hum Mol Genet. 2014.
31. Tyrrell JS, Whinney DJ, Ukoumunne OC, et al. Prevalence, associated factors, and comorbid conditions for Meniere's disease. Ear Hear. 2014;35:e162–9.
32. Frejo L, Soto-Varela A, Santos S, et al. Clinical subgroups in bilateral Meniere disease. Front Neurol. 2016;7:182.
33. Lempert T, Olesen J, Furman J, et al. Vestibular migraine: diagnostic criteria. J Vestib Res. 2012;22:167–72.
34. Derebery MJ. Allergic management of Meniere's disease: an outcome study. Otolaryngology Head Neck Surg. 2000;122:174–82.
35. Di Berardino F, Cesarani A. Gluten sensitivity in Meniere's disease. Laryngoscope. 2012;122:700–2.
36. Topuz B, Ogmen G, Ardic F, et al. Provocation of endolymphatic hydrops with a prick test in Meniere's disease. Adv Ther. 2007;24:819–25.
37. Keles E, et al. Meniere's disease and allergy: allergens and cytokines. J Laryngol Otol. 2004;118:688–93.
38. Fuse T, et al. Immunological responses in acute low-tone sensorineural hearing loss and Meniere's disease. Acta Otolaryngol. 2003;123:26–31.
39. Frejo L, et al. Proinflammatory cytokines and response to molds in mononuclear cells of patients with Meniere disease. Sci Rep. 2018;8:5974.1–11.
40. Naganawa S, Nakashima T. Visualization of endolymphatic hydrops with MR imaging in patients with Ménière's disease and related pathologies: current status of its methods and clinical significance. Jpn J Radiol. 2014;32(4):191–204.
41. Nakashima T, Naganawa S, Sugiura M, et al. Visualization of endolymphatic hydrops in patients with Meniere's disease. Laryngoscope. 2007;117:415–20.
42. Sepahdari AR, Ishiyama G, Vorasubin N, et al. Delayed intravenous contrast-enhanced 3D FLAIR MRI in Meniere's disease: correlation of quantitative measures of endolymphatic hydrops with hearing. Clin Imaging. 2015;39:26–31.
43. Jing Zou, Zhen Wang, Yukun Chen, et al. MRI detection of endolymphatic hydrops in Meniere's disease in 8 minutes using MIIRMR and a 20-channel coil after targeted gadolinium delivery. World J Otorhinolaryngol Head Neck Surg. 2019;5:180–7.
44. Radtke A, Lempert T, Gresty MA, et al. Migraine and Meniere's disease: is there a link? Neurology. 2002;59:1700–4.
45. Pyykko I, Manchaiah V, Farkkila M, et al. Association between Meniere's disease and vestibular migraine. Auris Nasus Larynx. 2019;46:724–33.
46. Ghavami Y, Mahboubi H, Yau AY, et al. Migraine features in patients with Meniere's disease. Laryngoscope. 2016;126(1):163–8.
47. Bruderer SG, Bodmer D, Stohler NA, et al. Population-based study on the epidemiology of Ménière's disease. Audiol Neurotol. 2017;22(2):74–82.
48. Swaminathan A, Smith JH. Migraine and vertigo. Curr Neurol Neurosci Rep. 2015;15(2):515.
49. Seo YJ, Kim J, Kim SH. The change of hippocampal volume and its relevance with inner ear function in Meniere's disease patients. Auris Nasus Larynx. 2016;43(6):620–5.
50. Wang Y, Diao T, Zhao Y, Yu L. The clinical characteristics and audiogram in 103 Meniere's disease patients with and without vestibular migraine. Clin Otolaryngol. 2017:1–4.
51. Nevoux J, et al. International consensus (ICON) on treatment of Ménière's disease. Eur Ann Otorhinolaryngol Head Neck Dis. 2018;135:S29–32.
52. Clinical Practice Guideline: Meniere's disease. Otolaryngol Head Neck Surg. 2020;162(2S):S1–55.
53. Rosenbaum A, Winter M. Is betahistine effective for Ménière's disease? Medwave. 2017;17(8):e7068.
54. Adrion C, Fischer CS, Wagner J, et al. BEMED Study Group. Efficacy and safety of betahistine treatment in patients with Meniere's disease: primary results of a long term, multicentre, double blind, randomised, placebo controlled, dose defining trial.
55. Lezius F, Adrion C, Mansmann U, et al. High-dosage Betahistine dihydrochloride between 288 and 480mg/day in patients with severe Ménière's disease: a case series. Eur Arch Otorrinolaringol. 2011;268:1237–40.

56. Huppert D, Strupp M, Brandt T. Long-term course of Meniere's disease revisited. Acta Otolaryngol. 2010;130(6):644–51.
57. House JW, Doherty JK, Fisher LM, et al. Meniere's disease: prevalence of contralateral ear involvement. Otol Neurotol. 2006;27(3):355–61.
58. Paparella MM, Mancini F. Trauma and Meniere's syndrome. Laryngoscope. 1983;93:1004–12.
59. Green JD Jr, Blum DJ, Harner SG. Longitudinal follow-up of patients with Meniere's disease. Otolaryngol Head Neck Surg. 1991;104(6):783–8.
60. Chaves AG, Boari L, Lei Munhoz MS. The outcome of patients with Menieres disease. Braz J Otorhinolaryngol. 2007;73(3):346–50.
61. Gazquez I, Soto-Varela A, Aran I, et al. High prevalence of systemic autoimmune diseases in patients with Menière's disease.
62. Lempert T, Neuhauser H. Epidemiology of vertigo, migraine and vestibular migraine. J Neurol. 2009;256:333–8.
63. Paparella MM. Benign paroxysmal positional vertigo and other vestibular symptoms in Meniere disease. Ear Nose Throat J. 2008;87:562.

Some Understanding of Vestibular Migraine

8

Jilei Zhang, Xingli Li, and Lisheng Yu

Dizziness is a symptom caused by multiple factors, and in recent years, there has been a deeper understanding of its etiology, particularly with significant advances in the treatment of benign paroxysmal positional vertigo. Another milestone achievement is the recognition of vestibular migraine (VM). The path to understanding this condition has been long and winding: from as early as 131 BC, when dizziness and headache were first linked as symptoms, to the establishment of affirmative VM and possible diagnostic criteria by the Barany Society in 2012 and its inclusion in the appendix of headache classifications by the International Headache Society in 2013. This international recognition solidified the existence of VM, with literature suggesting it as the leading disorder in episodic vestibular syndromes, possibly surpassing BPPV, warranting significant attention.

Domestically, attention to VM has grown in the past 2 years, with two versions of expert consensus published successively. Despite clear guidelines both domestically and internationally, the appropriate clinical application of these guidelines is not merely a matter of straightforward application but requires a thorough understanding of the disease and guidelines. Here, we present several current understandings of this disease stage, aiming to stimulate broader attention and accumulate more evidence.

J. Zhang · X. Li · L. Yu (✉)
Department of Otorhinolaryngology, Head and Neck Surgery, People's Hospital, Peking University, Beijing, China

8.1 Is Separate Research Necessary for the Treatment of Vestibular Migraine (VM), Given That Many Treatments Follow Migraine Guidelines?

Indeed, current versions of guidelines and consensus on VM list its diagnosis under migraine disorders and generally adhere to migraine treatment protocols. However, this does not negate the necessity of conducting independent research on VM; instead, it underscores the need for further investigation. Firstly, patients with VM present symptoms distinct from classical migraine, and in potential VM diagnoses, a history of (migraine) headache is not a prerequisite. Thus, these conditions may differ mechanistically from classical migraine, warranting specific research. Secondly, since their presentations and mechanisms may differ, treatments may also need to differ, though existing migraine treatment protocols can serve as a baseline. Comprehensive research from clinical and foundational aspects on the differences between VM and classical migraine is crucial to establishing whether VM is a subtype of migraine or an independent disease.

L. Yu (ed.), *Progress in Postauricular Administration*, Experts' Perspectives on Medical Advances,
https://doi.org/10.1007/978-981-95-5102-6_8

8.2 How Can Misdiagnosis and Underdiagnosis of VM Be Minimized?

Firstly, carefully interpreting existing VM guidelines is the crucial initial step to reduce underdiagnosis. However, understanding these guidelines can be confusing; unlike guidelines for conditions such as BPPV, which strictly define characteristics like nystagmus, or Meniere's disease, which specify attack forms and hearing loss criteria, VM diagnostic criteria lack specific symptom constraints. VM's clinical features are "variable," with diverse vestibular symptoms, attack durations, and forms, making it a chameleon in the realm of dizziness, capable of mimicking nearly all vestibular disorders. While guidelines for vestibular migraine do not define diagnostic features of the disease, they do affirm its existence. Some experts suggest this disease is somewhat elusive, and failure to acknowledge its existence could lead to significant underdiagnosis. Given the wide-ranging manifestations of VM, differential diagnosis is crucial, particularly since conditions easily confused with VM generally have relatively clear diagnostic criteria.

Therefore, the second critical step in diagnosing this disease is becoming familiar with standard criteria for other common causes of vertigo, thereby identifying discrepancies. This aspect will be elaborated in subsequent sections on distinguishing it from common diseases. Additionally, in diagnosing dizziness, a concept of "comorbidity" is essential; the diagnostic criteria for Meniere's disease, benign paroxysmal positional vertigo, and VM operate at different levels, making it entirely possible for the same patient to experience them concurrently or sequentially. Furthermore, in the diagnosis of dizziness, a dynamic perspective is necessary; distinguishing between dizziness diseases is challenging at the onset, but as the condition progresses and recurs, unique features may emerge. Therefore, interventions at different time points may lead to varied diagnoses, a consideration worth noting in clinical practice.

8.3 Differentiation and Comorbidity Between Vestibular Migraine (VM) and Meniere's Disease (MD) [1]

The pathogenesis of Meniere's disease involves endolymphatic hydrops, although autopsy findings indicate that the occurrence rate of hydrops can reach up to 6%, whereas the prevalence of Meniere's disease itself is only 0.2%. Despite excellent animal models for endolymphatic hydrops, there is currently no model for the rupture of the membranous labyrinth in Meniere's disease. Meniere's disease is a clinical syndrome characterized by spontaneous episodic vertigo, fluctuating sensorineural hearing loss, tinnitus, and aural fullness (the tetrad). However, only 50% of patients initially present with both vertigo and hearing loss, 19% solely with vertigo, and 26% solely with hearing loss. It is generally believed that the tetrad should appear 3–5 years after onset, with progressive hearing loss in Meniere's disease evolving from fluctuating low-frequency hearing loss to severe flat-type deafness over this period. Hearing tests are crucial in differentiating MD from VM. In addition, patients with pure MD typically keep their eyes open during vertigo attacks (visual compensation), while VM patients avoid visual stimuli and keep their eyes closed. When VM coexists with MD, symptoms may lessen with closed eyes but dizziness persists. Vertigo in isolated VM often completely disappears with closed eyes.

Furthermore, the frequency of attacks differs between the two conditions. The pathogenesis of Meniere's disease involves endolymphatic hydrops, where symptoms appear only when the hydrops reaches a critical point of rupture. The generation and worsening of hydrops to the point of rupture take time, and repeated occurrences over a short period are unlikely. Studies show that patients with MD and affirmed VM have an average of 7.1 attacks per month, those with possible VM have 4 attacks per month, and patients with pure MD have 1.6 attacks per month. Therefore, frequent and repetitive attacks, even daily occurrences, almost certainly exclude pure Meniere's disease and suggest a diagnosis of at least concomitant vestibular migraine. Another distinguishing factor is electronystagmography (ENG). During MD attacks, there are distinct peripheral pathological nystagmus characteristics, while during VM attacks and interictal periods, mild central and peripheral pathological nystagmus may appear, with predominantly mild central pathological nystagmus.

Apart from differentiation between the two, it is essential to note the possibility of comorbidity between MD and VM. As early as 1861, Meniere mentioned headache among patients. The incidence of different types of headaches among Meniere's disease patients can reach 70–76%, with migraine incidence ranging from 22% to 56%. Patients with characteristics of both Meniere's disease and vestibular migraine (Migraine-Meniere's disease, MMD) have been reported multiple times. Studies indicate that 64.1% of MD patients have affirmed or possible VM. Such a high comorbidity rate between the two may indicate different manifestations under the same mechanism or a possible causal relationship. Inner ear MRI studies show that 21% of VM patients with auditory symptoms have endolymphatic hydrops, suggesting that migraine mechanisms may contribute to the occurrence of membranous labyrinth hydrops. Therefore, in at least some cases of Meniere's disease, there may be a relationship with migraine mechanisms. Some literature even suggests that 95% of MD patients exhibit different migraine symptoms, potentially classifying MD as a special type of VM. This viewpoint is somewhat radical, considering that besides migraine, many factors can influence the onset of Meniere's disease, such as immune factors, trauma, acute otitis media, labyrinthitis, and anatomical variations in the inner ear.

However, as proposed by the European Meniere's Classification, there is a type of Meniere's disease associated with migraine, characterized by a younger age of onset and a significantly higher incidence of bilateral onset. Treatment strategies should combine antimigraine therapies while avoiding destructive treatments to prevent bilateral vestibular function impairment or loss. Inner ear-related Meniere's disease can follow a stepwise treatment plan, with corresponding therapies administered (see Chap. 7).

8.4 Differentiation and Comorbidity Between Vestibular Migraine (VM) and Benign Paroxysmal Positional Vertigo (BPPV)

Benign paroxysmal positional vertigo (BPPV) and migraine are both common vestibular disorders. BPPV results from displaced otoliths in the semicircular canals or otolithic organs, characterized by typical nystagmus features and manifestations. However, among patients exhibiting positional nystagmus, only 40.5% meet the diagnostic criteria for BPPV (see Chap. 14). A significant proportion of VM patients also experience positional nystagmus, with distinct differences in nystagmus characteristics. The most common positional nystagmus in VM is low-frequency, low-velocity persistent nystagmus, predominantly horizontal and persistent, occasionally presenting other types of mild persistent nystagmus. Secondly, the frequency of attacks differs significantly between the two conditions. BPPV typically recurs once a year or every few years, with each episode lasting several weeks before resolving, whereas VM can recur within months, with each episode lasting 2–3 days before improvement. Thirdly, the efficacy of repositioning maneuvers differs between VM and BPPV. Repositioning maneuvers for BPPV are ineffective in treating positional vertigo associated with migraine. Additionally, caution is necessary during repositioning maneuvers to avoid triggering migraine attacks due to patient anxiety and severe dizziness. Finally, the demographic of affected individuals also differs: BPPV primarily affects individuals aged 50–60 years, whereas those with positional vertigo due to BPPV tend to be younger, aged 40–50 years. Suspicion of VM rather than pure BPPV should be raised in cases presenting with recurrent attacks, episodes lasting 2–3 days, age 30–40 years, low-frequency, low-velocity persistent nystagmus, and absence of alternating nystagmus.

The coccurrence rate of BPPV and VM is high. BPPV is merely a symptomatic diagnosis. What causes the displacement of otoliths?

Inner ear blood supply, calcium metabolism abnormalities, and inner ear diseases such as VM and MD can all cause otolith displacement. The higher incidence of BPPV in females around the age of 50 is related to menopausal calcium metabolism changes and the higher prevalence of migraine among female patients. Patients with a history of migraine have a threefold higher incidence of BPPV compared to those without a history of migraine, which is a well-established risk factor. Therefore, in the spectrum of dizziness disorders, BPPV, VM, and psychosomatic-related disorders cannot be strictly separated into distinct categories based solely on incidence rates; they interact in a circular relationship, potentially cooccurring in the same patient or appearing consecutively.

8.5 Vestibular Neuritis and VM

Vestibular neuritis is a benign self-limiting disease within acute vestibular syndrome, classified into two types in textbooks: single episode and multiple recurring episodes. This recurrent type refers to repeated episodes of vertigo without accompanying hearing loss. In 2020, experts reached a consensus that vestibular neuritis rarely recurs; once recurrence occurs, this diagnosis is no longer considered. This recurrent type of isolated vertigo resembles the vestibular type described in Meniere's criteria from 1972, suggesting that vestibular-type Meniere's may more closely align with the diagnosis of vestibular migraine.

Vestibular neuritis is a self-limiting disease; initial vertigo is severe, gradually easing with static compensation, but subsequent motion-induced dizziness can persist for a long time and requires extended recovery time for dynamic compensation. VM can also cause rotary vertigo, but symptoms can resolve quickly. Secondly, during attacks, the eye movement manifestations of the two conditions differ; vestibular neuritis exhibits typical peripheral vestibular nystagmus, whereas in most cases of VM, nystagmus is not prominent, indicating a separation of symptoms and signs.

8.6 Vestibular Paroxysmia and VM

Vestibular paroxysmia has a single mechanism of onset, leading to consistent manifestations regardless of the frequency of attacks, characterized by stereotyped attacks. VM, however, has multiple mechanisms of onset and variable symptoms, marking the most crucial differentiation between the two. When differentiation is challenging, both conditions may be treated with antiepileptic drugs without causing significant disruption during treatment.

8.7 What to Do with a Large Number of Paroxysmal Vertigo Syndromes That Do Not Meet Current Diagnostic Criteria?

Considering that Meniere's disease may initially present with isolated vertigo or cochlear symptoms, in 1972, guidelines classified Meniere's disease into cochlear-type and vestibular-type, but many cases of cochlear-type or vestibular-type Meniere's do not progress to typical Meniere's tetrad. Although vestibular-type Meniere's and vestibular migraine are closely related, a significant portion of patients with paroxysmal vestibular syndromes do not meet current diagnostic criteria, including BPPV, MD, and VM. How should they be treated? Guidelines summarize scientific norms based on existing evidence, yet treating diseases is an art, especially when dealing with individual heterogeneity. Although these patients can currently only be diagnosed with benign recurrent vertigo (BRV), clinical consideration must take into account the high prevalence of migraine predisposition in the general population. Recent literature has continuously observed BRV groups, which show similarities in age to VM, older than MD, with a higher proportion of females similar to VM, more pronounced than MD. Hence, providing antimigraine treatment may be most suitable for these patients at this stage.

Headache is a symptom, and migraine is a pathogenic mechanism, currently considered a reversible brain functional disorder. Within this pathogenic mechanism, manifestations without headache symptoms are entirely possible, such as abdominal migraine in current migraine classifications, benign recurrent vertigo in children. Viewing migraine from a developmental perspective, as a brain disease, its manifestations can be systemic. Therefore, in diagnosing this disease, a multidisciplinary approach is required to view disease manifestations in different systems under the same pathological mechanism. Individuals with different migraine predispositions may exhibit completely different manifestations at different times; headache, dizziness, deafness, tinnitus, and diarrhea may all be personalized symptoms of migraine without necessarily having headache.

8.8 How to Understand Chronic Vestibular Migraine?

VM has a high incidence rate, being the most common episodic vestibular syndrome disease, capable of mimicking clinical features of all other episodic vestibular syndrome diseases. However, VM guideline 3.11 also mentions the possibility of chronic VM as a disease type, with a significant correlation between acute vertigo chronicization and anxiety. The proportion of migraines accompanied by psychological disorders can be as high as 65%. VM's repetitive attacks continuously impact the central vestibular compensation system and emotional system, easily leading to manifestations of chronic dizziness. Some scholars have proposed the concept of MARD (migraine anxiety-related dizziness). Whether chronic VM is an independent disease type or comorbid with psychogenic dizziness remains inconclusive. However, when diagnosing chronic vestibular syndrome, VM's role in its pathogenesis should be considered, not entirely placing it within the diagnostic system of episodic vestibular syndromes.

8.9 Patient Education Is the Most Important First Step in Treating VM

For chronic diseases with a genetic predisposition and recurring attacks that are difficult to cure completely, both lifestyle and drug management are essential, with lifestyle management being more important. For this disease, patient education is crucial, ensuring correct understanding and avoiding triggers is vital in controlling disease attacks.

Firstly, how to perceive migraine? This population has a highly sensitive brain, capable of perceiving things that a normal brain cannot, serving as a protective mechanism, helping individuals avoid risks. On the other hand, excessive stimulation can harm the brain, such as excessive fatigue, staying up late, and excessive emotional burdens, potentially triggering migraine occurrences, necessitating stopping to rest and halt behaviors detrimental to health. Therefore, for the body, it is protective; some scholars believe that the migraine mechanism is an evolutionary advantage for humans.

Additionally, avoiding triggers is essential. Migraine occurrence is related to diet, sleep, emotions, hormone levels, atmospheric pressure, and more. However, patients must understand that migraine occurrence is the result of multiple factors acting together. Thus, understanding this disease well and self-management are crucial. Advising patients to avoid all possible risk factors is not always feasible. Once, a female patient revisited me and said she did not sleep well last night and was especially worried about having an attack. Hearing this, I reflected on my patient education not being entirely successful and explained again to the patient that the disease's occurrence is due to the accumulation of multiple triggering factors reaching a threshold. Therefore, if only a single triggering factor is present, it often does not cause illness. Relaxing mentally is more critical. Hearing these words, the patient relaxed. After all, the triggers of migraine are numerous; clothing, food, shelter, and climate are unavoidable factors. Excessive worry among patients may promote triggering.

8.10 How to Manage Drug Treatment During the Acute Phase?

Regarding treatment during the acute phase, clinical research is relatively scarce. Some studies suggest that calcium channel blockers are effective. A study utilized randomized, double-blind crossover, placebo-controlled methods with 73 patients, randomly divided into 2 groups: the zonisamide group (2.5 mg) and the placebo group. Symptom recording was done using structured diaries, with the main study endpoint being the improvement from moderate to severe vertigo to mild or none after 2 h of medication (treatment effectiveness). Analysis of data from 10 patients (17 episodes of VM attacks) showed that the proportion of patients with effective treatment of vertigo after 2 h was 38% in the zonisamide group (95% CI; 9–76), compared to 22% in the placebo group (95% CI; 3–60) (Neuhauser H, 2003). However, our hospital does not have such drugs and lacks experience in their use. Currently, symptomatic treatments such as promethazine are mainly used in clinical practice, with most patients showing significant improvement after rest. However, from a pathogenic perspective, NSAIDs and calcium channel blockers should be effective during the acute phase of migraine. Hospitals with the capacity may consider trying these medications to accumulate more experience and evidence. As mentioned earlier, although currently treated similarly to migraine, VM should be considered as an independent disease with different pathogenic mechanisms, thus requiring specific treatment emphasis, which we hope will be supported by better evidence in future research.

8.11 Drug Management in Preventive Therapy: Who Should Use It and How?

8.11.1 Indications for Preventive Therapy

Not all patients require preventive medication. Consider preventive therapy if one of the following conditions applies: (1) long duration of attacks or disability caused by attacks, (2) poor response to acute phase treatment, (3) monthly frequency of attacks exceeding three times (typically $\geq$ 2 times for migraine), and (4) patient request for treatment. Although specific numbers are not available, clinically, vestibular migraine attacks appear less frequent than migraine, occurring once every 1–2 months or even several months. It is generally recommended that patients take medication for 2 weeks after an attack, to aid rapid recovery and stabilize disrupted vestibular function, thereby raising the threshold and preventing repeated attacks due to a lower threshold, excessive anxiety, and entering a vicious cycle of attacks. For those with particularly frequent attacks, medication for prevention is considered every 1–2 weeks.

8.11.2 Course of Preventive Medication

In literature reports, the observation of efficacy generally begins at the third month of treatment, with many studies observing efficacy between 3 and 6 months. There are currently no recommendations for the course of preventive treatment for VM, both domestically and abroad. Based on the criteria for evaluating efficacy, the typical course of preventive treatment for migraine is generally 6 months (see Table 8.1).

Table 8.1 Criteria for assessing the effectiveness of preventive medication (Expert Consensus on Diagnosis and Treatment of Vestibular Migraine (2018))

Assessment items		
Visual analog scale	No symptoms (0 points)—maximum possible dizziness (10 points)	
Severity of symptom	Very mild	1 point
	Mild	2 points
	Moderate	3 points
	Severe	4 points
	Very severe	5 points
Duration of attacks	Evaluated in hours	–
Frequency of attacks	High frequency (1–4 points)	1 point: >5 times per week 2 points: 3–4 times per week 3 points: Once per week 4 points: 2–3 times per month
	Low frequency (5–6 points)	5 points: 2–3 times every 3 months 6 points: <2 times every 3 months
Evaluation of efficacy	Improved (0–2 points)	0 points: No improvement 1 point: Slight improvement 2 points: Moderate improvement
	Significant improvement (3–4 points)	3 points: significant improvement 4 points: symptoms disappeared

8.11.3 Preventive Medication

Currently, preventive medication for VM follows that of migraine. Here, I will discuss my own experience with medication:

The pathogenesis of migraine is currently unclear, and many medications can be effective, including numerous traditional Chinese medicines, which may also benefit certain patients. Therefore, preventive medication in clinical practice can be highly flexible and individualized. Encouraging patients to explore their own experiences with medication is crucial, as this disease cannot be eradicated. Finding effective methods for oneself can greatly alleviate disease-related anxiety.

Since it is recommended in guidelines, the efficacy of medications is self-evident. Therefore, more attention should be paid to the side effects of medications. For example, topiramate may exacerbate depression and cause extrapyramidal symptoms, so it should be used with caution in patients with depression and the elderly. Amitriptyline may affect appetite and may be more suitable for young women concerned with appearance. Valproate may induce polycystic ovary syndrome, so women of childbearing age should be cautious. Gabapentin is relatively safe, but a small number of patients may experience severe dizziness after use. Antiepileptic drugs are preferably not used as first-line treatments, as many patients are deterred from using them after reading the package inserts, greatly reducing patient compliance. When prescribing medication, careful consideration should be given to patients' accompanying symptoms. Patients with sleep and mood disorders should avoid using topiramate; better results may be achieved with antianxiety and antidepressant medications.

Literature mentions that when patients report significant auditory symptoms such as tinnitus, acetazolamide is the preferred choice; acetazolamide and lamotrigine are suitable for refractory patients, with acetazolamide showing more significant effects in reducing the frequency and severity of dizziness and headache attacks (Zhao Yue, Current Research on Vestibular Migraine, 2019).

Most drugs recommended for migraine require dose adjustments and course controls; patients who cannot attend follow-up visits on time should use medications cautiously.

Personally, I use a variety of medications such as topiramate, gabapentin, amitriptyline, flunarizine, and duloxetine. For infrequent attacks, occurring once every 1–2 months or even every few months, I administer topiramate for 2 weeks after an attack. For frequent attacks, occurring

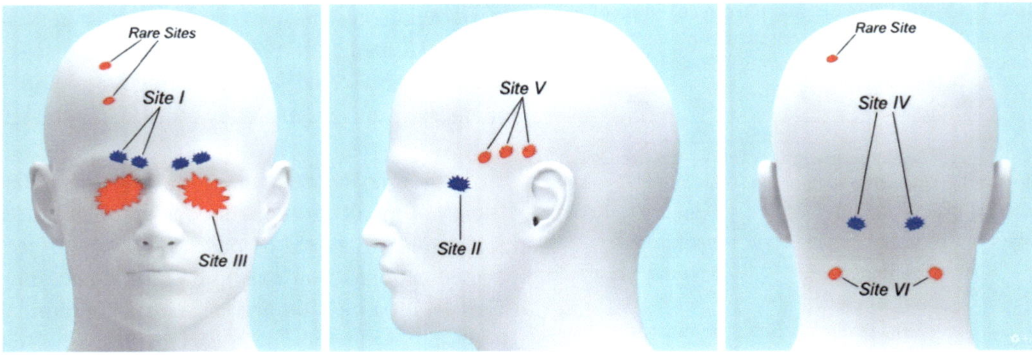

Fig. 8.1 Common sites of nerve entrapment

once every 1–2 weeks, I prescribe different medications based on the situation. These patients often have an urgent desire for treatment to quickly stabilize their attacks. Gabapentin works faster than amitriptyline, so I generally prefer gabapentin, especially as a second-line treatment for menopausal symptoms, making it my initial choice for menopausal women experiencing repeated dizziness. Flunarizine and duloxetine are used in combination based on patient mood assessments. For those needing rapid relief, I start with flunarizine, while for those with poor emotional states requiring longer adjustment times, I directly use duloxetine. It is important to note that patients exhibit significant individual differences in their responses to medications. Pharmacology guides medication use, but ultimately, the patient's response to the medication should determine its use.

8.11.4 Nonpharmacological Treatment

There are numerous neuromodulation therapies mentioned in the literature for migraine, which have shown good efficacy and can be used for patients who refuse medication or have frequent attacks. One such product introduced domestically is Cefaly, an external trigeminal nerve stimulation device (e-TNS) that delivers precise micropulses to the ophthalmic branch of the trigeminal nerve via electrodes placed on the forehead to treat migraines.

8.11.5 Surgical Treatment

(1) PFO closure: Patent foramen ovale (PFO) closure is a high-risk factor for migraines. After closure, some patients experience relief from headaches. This approach can also be considered for VM patients.
(2) Neurovascular decompression surgery: This surgical procedure originated from cosmetic surgery patients experiencing reduced migraine attacks postoperatively. However, there is limited research on its effectiveness for vestibular migraine.

The nerves often irritated by compression include supraorbital nerve, supratrochlear nerve, zygomatic-temporal nerve, greater occipital nerve, etc. (see Fig. 8.1). Operation should be performed according to the different conformity of point and conformity of nature, for individual muscles cut, bone tube mill, or nerve isolation. Usually done under local anesthesia, the operation is relatively simple, about 30–40 min; routine preoperative examination of qualified patients and perioperative risk is relatively small.

(3) In addition to the two surgical methods widely recognized in the literature, endolymphatic sac decompression surgery also plays a role in preventing migraine and VM attacks. There is a bidirectional impact between migraines and the inner ear; migraine attacks can affect the inner ear, leading to dizziness caused by repeated ruptures of the inner ear membrane labyrinth, which can also trigger migraine attacks. Removing the inner ear stimulus has a certain effect on preventing migraine and VM attacks.

Reference

1. Yu L, Si F, Ma X, et al. Meniere Disease and vestibular migraine [J]. J Clin Otorhinolaryngol Head Neck Surg. 2016;30(12):925–7.

9 Sudden Sensorineural Hearing Loss

Yuanyuan Jing, Qi Liu, and Lisheng Yu

9.1 Definition of Sudden Deafness

Sudden sensorineural hearing loss (SSNHL), also known as idiopathic sudden sensorineural hearing loss (ISSNHL), is a common emergency in the field of otolaryngology. According to the Chinese Medical Association's Guidelines for the Diagnosis and Treatment of Sudden Deafness (2015), sudden deafness is defined as "sudden, unexplained sensorineural hearing loss that occurs within 72 hours, with a decrease in hearing of at least 20 dBHL at two adjacent frequencies."

The definition of sudden sensorineural hearing loss (SSNHL) includes three important points. Firstly, the cause has not been identified. Once the cause is identified, it is no longer diagnosed as SSNHL, as at that time, SSNHL is just a symptom of the disease. Secondly, it is defined as sensorineural hearing loss, characterized by a decrease in hearing of over 20 dB at two adjacent frequencies. Additionally, the onset occurs within 72 h and reaches a peak within 3 days. It is important to note that "unexplained" does not mean there is no cause; it simply reflects the current limitations of our understanding. All diseases have causes, including tinnitus, which has complex causes, but that does not mean it has no cause.

Y. Jing · Q. Liu · L. Yu (✉)
Department of Otorhinolaryngology, Head and Neck Surgery, People's Hospital, Peking University, Beijing, China
e-mail: 1710301140@pku.edu.cn

9.2 Classification of SSNHL

SSNHL is categorized into high-frequency hearing loss, low-frequency hearing loss, flat-type hearing loss, and total deafness (including profound deafness) based on the frequency and severity of the hearing impairment. Different types of hearing loss may have different underlying causes. High-frequency hearing loss may result from damage to the outer hair cells (up to 50 dB of hearing loss) or inner hair cells (at least 60 dB of hearing loss). The primary cause of low-frequency hearing loss may be endolymphatic hydrops or local blood supply disorders affecting the cochlear spiral ligament, resulting in tissue damage due to hypoxia and electrolyte imbalance. Flat type is primarily attributed to functional disorders of the inner ear vascular plexus and/or cochlear vascular supply, as well as tissue hypoxia. Currently, total deafness or near-total deafness, such as profound deafness, is believed to be caused by vascular embolism or thrombosis of the cochlear artery or modiolar artery. Migraine is currently considered to be one of the significant causes of sudden deafness and can present as various types of hearing loss.

L. Yu (ed.), *Progress in Postauricular Administration*, Experts' Perspectives on Medical Advances,
https://doi.org/10.1007/978-981-95-5102-6_9

9.2.1 Low-Frequency Descending Type

The main pathological and physiological mechanism may be endolymphatic hydrops. In clinical practice, it has the highest recovery rate, with a recovery rate up to 78.16%. Some literature reports a self-healing rate of over 50%. In the 1985 American Meniere's disease treatment guidelines, a cochlear type of Meniere's disease was identified, which corresponds to this classification. However, in 1995, this classification was removed from the guidelines for Meniere's disease. While both conditions have the pathological basis of endolymphatic hydrops, the severity varies. Endolymphatic hydrops is not limited to Meniere's disease; other inner ear conditions can also result in endolymphatic hydrops. In Western countries, postmortem examinations have revealed that 6% of people have endolymphatic hydrops, regardless of symptoms. However, only 0.2% of people have a history of Meniere's disease, making it 30 times less common. This indicates that endolymphatic hydrops and Meniere's disease cannot be equated. Endolymphatic hydrops is a common pathological condition linked to various diseases, including low-frequency sensorineural hearing loss, fluctuating low-frequency sensorineural hearing loss, including Meniere's disease, vestibular migraine, and certain systemic conditions that result in low-frequency hearing loss, such as autoimmune inner ear disease and hypothyroidism. All of these factors can lead to endolymphatic hydrops. In addition, low-frequency sensorineural hearing loss is likely to be confused with cochlear migraine and may be a variant of it.

9.2.2 Flat Type

Sudden deafness of the flat type primarily involves the functional impairment of the inner ear blood vessels and/or obstruction of blood supply of the cochlea, resulting in tissue hypoxia. Flat-type SSNHL is defined as a decrease in hearing across all frequencies, with an average hearing threshold of ≤80 dBHL at 500, 1000, 2000, and 4000 Hz. According to a national multicenter study on SSNHL, the recovery rate for flat-type SSNHL is 34.58%, and the effective rate is 82.59%, second to low-frequency descending type. In a reclassification of sudden deafness by Ma Xin, the flat type SSNHL was further categorized. Based on the disparity in air-conduction thresholds at 1000 Hz and 4000 Hz, differences exceeding 15 dB were classified as either ascending or descending type SSNHL, while differences within 15 dB were defined as consistent type SSNHL. The results indicated that the prognosis for the ascending type of SSNHL with a flat curve is relatively better. However, there were no statistically significant differences between the descending type, consistent type, and total deafness, suggesting a correlation between hearing prognosis and curve type. The study suggests that SSNHL classified as ascending type, which includes the low-frequency descending type, flat type, and total deafness ascending type as proposed in the guidelines, may have a better prognosis. The main pathogenic mechanism is believed to be varying degrees of hydrops or vascular arterial disease. On the other hand, the descending type includes the high-frequency descending type and flat type, as well as total deafness descending-type SSNHL as proposed in the guidelines. The main pathology involves hair cell damage and is associated with a poorer prognosis. Flat consistent type and total deafness type may be related to obstruction of blood supply and potential labyrinthitis, leading to a poorer prognosis.

9.2.3 Profound Deafness Type

Profound or near-total deafness may be caused by vascular occlusion or thrombosis of the cochlear artery or the labyrinthine artery. An average hearing threshold of >80 dBHL at 500, 1000, 2000, and 4000 Hz is defined as profound deafness. The recovery rate for profound deafness is the lowest, at only 14.49%, with many cases being of the ascending type. Clinical reports and practices have shown that enhancing circulation in the inner ear, reducing blood viscosity, and using anticoagulant thrombolytic therapy can significantly improve hearing. Moreover, most studies indicate a significant increase in plasma fibrinogen levels in patients with SSNHL compared to the control group. However, the cure rate and effectiveness of treatment for profound deafness are currently low, indicating the potential presence of other underlying disease mechanisms.

Profoundly deaf individuals should consider the possibility of cochlear neuritis. While facial neuritis and vestibular neuritis are well known, the existence of cochlear neuritis is not yet supported by clear diagnostic criteria.

In cases of inner ear bleeding, 3D-FLAIR MRI can be utilized to assess labyrinthine lesions in patients experiencing SSNHL. Abnormal high signal in the inner ear suggests the possibility of inner ear bleeding, often accompanied by dizziness, severe hearing loss, and mostly profound deafness, with poor chances of recovery. If inner ear bleeding is confirmed as the clear cause, it cannot be diagnosed as SSNHL, as sudden hearing loss and dizziness are just symptoms of inner ear bleeding. In addition, when examining the inner ear with MRI, the presence of high-density shadows in the inner ear may have various other causes, such as localized labyrinthitis, which can exhibit similar MRI findings. Therefore, additional evidence is required to confirm the presence of inner ear bleeding.

9.2.4 High-Frequency Descending Type

High-frequency hearing loss may result from damage to the outer hair cells (up to 50 dB of hearing loss) or inner hair cells (at least 60 dB of hearing loss). The recovery and effectiveness rates for treatment are only slightly higher than those for complete deafness. The therapeutic effect for patients with a flat, total deafness, or descending type curve is also not optimal. In a study by Li Shuijing and colleagues, it was found that the levels of fibrinogen in patients with high-frequency descending type significantly increased at the onset of the disease. This suggests that the onset of the disease may be influenced by factors related to microcirculation disorders in the vestibular cochlear branch. In future clinical studies, it is necessary to consider the addition of fibrinolytic drugs for the treatment of SSNHL with high-frequency descending type.

9.3 SSNHL Accompanied by Tinnitus

Eighty percent of cases of SSNHL are accompanied by varying degrees of tinnitus. When SSNHL occurs, the inner ear experiences sudden damage, leading to an abrupt change in sound information that signals the brain. The brain actively compensates for the hearing loss, while the tinnitus serves as a reminder to the patient. The tinnitus that accompanies SSNHL is a manifestation of the brain's alertness. When SSNHL sets in, a certain level of tinnitus can serve as a clear reminder to the patient of the presence of a pathological condition. Research by Ma Xin and colleagues found that there is no clear relationship between the degree of hearing loss and the intensity of tinnitus. Regardless of the degree of hearing loss, tinnitus intensity is typically concentrated at levels 3–4. On one hand, tinnitus can activate the body's emotional and sympathetic nervous systems, thereby enhancing the body's compensatory efficiency for hearing loss. On the other hand, it does not have a significant impact on the patient. This suggests that tinnitus may serve as a protective mechanism of the body and is generally not considered particularly severe, unless the patient has certain susceptibility factors or is in an anxious state. This is particularly evident in female patients over the age of 45, where the prevalence of level 4 tinnitus is significantly higher in female patients over 45 than in male patients. Given that 45 is typically the onset of menopause in women, the decrease in estrogen's protective impact on the auditory system, along with fluctuations in estrogen levels, can modify the brain's receptor sensitivity to 5-HT, which is crucial in the emotional system. Another phenomenon to note is that during the treatment of SSNHL, a sudden worsening of tinnitus and sound aversion is not necessarily negative. It often indicates a sign of hearing recovery, typically occurring when the hearing recovers to around 60 dB. Understanding this phenomenon is crucial for guiding medication and boosting patients' confidence in their recovery.

9.4 SSNHL Accompanied by Dizziness

Around 30% of patients with SSNHL also experience varying degrees of dizziness, which could manifest as lightheadedness, vertigo, or unsteadiness. Vertigo can present as brief episodes resembling benign paroxysmal positional vertigo (BPPV), or as prolonged episodes, each with distinct characteristics.

Therefore, it is crucial to carefully analyze and assess the situation. If benign paroxysmal positional vertigo occurs after SSNHL, it typically does not occur on the same day as the onset of SSNHL. The onset of symptoms typically occurs a few days later because the initial response to inner ear ischemia during SSNHL causes the dislodgement of ear stones into the semicircular canals. This process takes time to occur and does not happen simultaneously with SSNHL. If the patient experiences a sudden onset of vertigo, similar to benign paroxysmal positional vertigo (BPPV), it typically has minimal impact on the prognosis of hearing. However, patients experiencing prolonged and continuous vertigo often have a poorer prognosis. Additionally, some patients experience lightheadedness, which has multifaceted causes and often involves the central nervous system. This may be due to insufficient cerebral blood supply or a state of cerebral congestion. Furthermore, in patients with complete deafness, they often complain of a sensation of their ears feeling "dead," accompanied by a feeling of fullness and loss of sensation around the ears. During the treatment process, sensation around the ears often recovers before hearing improvement.

The abnormal vestibular function in patients with SSNHL indicates a wide range and severe degree of inner ear damage. The video head impulse test (vHIT) can qualitatively and quantitatively analyze the damage to the three semicircular canals, while vestibular-evoked myogenic potentials can assess the function of the utricle and saccule. Studies have shown that the prevalence of abnormal function in the posterior semicircular canals is highest among patients with SSNHL and dizziness, possibly due to the blood supply to the inner ear. The internal auditory artery branches into the cochlear artery, which further divides into the cochlear branch and the vestibulocochlear branch. The latter mainly supplies the basal turn of the cochlea, the ampulla of the posterior semicircular canal, and most of the saccule. However, vestibular function testing has certain limitations. For instance, the caloric test can only evaluate the ultra-low-frequency function of the horizontal semicircular canal, and any irregularity along the entire testing pathway can result in abnormal findings.

9.5 Diagnosis of SSNHL

Diagnosing SSNHL must first rule out serious conditions such as stroke, nasopharyngeal cancer, acoustic neuroma, and metastasis of systemic tumors. Clinically, it is essential to prioritize addressing life-threatening conditions rather than focusing solely on the localized issue of hearing loss. Unilateral deafness is typically caused by a local lesion, while bilateral deafness necessitates consideration of systemic issues such as autoimmune diseases and endocrine disorders.

9.6 Treatment of SSNHL

In the treatment of SSNHL, the "Guidelines for Diagnosis and Treatment of SSNHL" (2015) emphasize the use of a classification-based approach based on the audiogram. There is a strong correlation between treatment outcomes and classification. The low-frequency type shows the best treatment efficacy, followed by the flat type, while the high-frequency drop type and total deafness type demonstrate poorer outcomes. Additionally, it is observed that most cases in the acute phase are caused by vascular disorders in the inner ear. Therefore, the recommended treatment involves the use of glucocorticoids in combination with a hemorheological drug to enhance microcirculation in the inner ear. The combined use of drugs targeting inner ear microcirculation and glucocorticoids is more effective than using a single therapy.

9.6.1 Use of Glucocorticoids

Glucocorticoid (GC) refers to the naturally occurring cortisol, also known as hydrocortisone, which is primarily produced in the human body. In healthy adults, the daily secretion of glucocorticoids ranges from 15 to 25 mg, and it exerts a wide range of effects in the body. Pharmacological doses of glucocorticoids mainly exhibit antiinflammatory, immunosuppressive, and antishock properties. However, while suppressing inflammation and alleviating symptoms, glucocorticoids also compromise the body's defense mechanisms, leading to increased susceptibility to infections and impaired wound healing. Therefore, in clinical practice, the rational use of glucocorticoids is essential. The physiological secretion pattern of glucocorticoids shows an increase starting from 2 to 4 am, reaching its peak between 8 and 10 am, and decreasing to the lowest level at 24:00.

9.6.1.1 Common Glucocorticoid Medications

Glucocorticoid medications can be classified into short-acting, intermediate-acting, and long-acting steroids based on their duration of biological effects. Short-acting steroids, such as prednisone and hydrocortisone, are natural hormones with weak antiinflammatory potency and short duration of action. They are not suitable for the treatment of SSNHL and are mainly used as replacement therapy for adrenal insufficiency. Intermediate-acting steroids are synthetic hormones and include dexamethasone, prednisolone, methylprednisolone, and deflazacort. Long-acting steroids, such as dexamethasone and betamethasone, are also synthetic hormones. Dexamethasone has strong antiinflammatory potency and a long duration of action but exhibits significant suppression of the hypothalamic-pituitary-adrenal (HPA) axis, making it unsuitable for long-term use. Betamethasone is primarily used for local administration, and the commonly used formulation is betamethasone dipropionate. In the treatment of SSNHL, commonly used medications are usually intermediate-acting and long-acting glucocorticoids, including prednisone, methylprednisolone, dexamethasone, and betamethasone.

For information on the equivalent doses, antiinflammatory potency, receptor affinity, half-life, duration of action, water and sodium retention potency, and HPA axis suppression duration of commonly used glucocorticoids, please refer to Table 9.1. The selection of the optimal medication and dosage based on the characteristics of each drug and different routes of administration will be discussed in detail in the following sections.

9.6.1.2 Advantages and Disadvantages of Different Routes of Glucocorticoid Administration

Glucocorticoids are first-line drugs for the treatment of SSNHL and can be administered systemically or locally. Local administration includes intratympanic administration and retroauricular administration.

(1) *Systemic administration* is currently the standard treatment approach for SSNHL. However, when administered systemically, the drugs must pass through the blood-labyrinth barrier in the inner ear to reach their site of action, resulting in insufficient effective drug concentration in the inner ear. Systemic administration may also cause side effects such as blood pressure and blood sugar fluctuations, gastrointestinal ulcers, etc., which limits its use in patients with underlying conditions like diabetes and hypertension.
(2) *Intratympanic administration* is a commonly used local administration route in clinical practice. It allows small molecules such as glucocorticoids to bypass the blood-labyrinth barrier and enter the inner ear, maintaining a higher concentration of drugs in the inner ear. Intratympanic administration also reduces many of the side effects associated with systemic administration. The Chinese guidelines recommend intratympanic administration as a salvage therapy when systemic administration is not feasible. However, intratympanic administration is an invasive treatment and has its drawbacks, including the risk of middle ear infection, drug loss

Table 9.1 Comparison table of commonly used glucocorticoids

Category	Common name	Name of ingredient	Antiinflammatory equivalent dose(mg)	Strength of antiinflammatory action	Receptor affinity	Plasma half-life (min)	Duration of action (h)	Strength of HPA axis inhibition	Duration of HPA axis inhibition (days)	Hydro-sodium storage
Moderate-acting	Prednisone	Prednisone	5	4	5	60	12–36	4	1.25–1.50	0.8
	Methylprednisolone	Methylprednisolone	4	5	1190	180	12–36	5	1.25–1.50	0.5
Long-acting	Dexamethasone	Dexamethasone	0.75	25	710	100–300	36–54	50	2.75	0
	Betamethasone	Betamethasone	0.6	25	540	100–300	36–54	50	3.25	0

through the eustachian tube, difficulties in controlling the dosage reaching the inner ear, and inconsistent sustained drug effects.

(3) *Retroauricular administration* is a safe, convenient, and minimally invasive new administration method that our research team has discovered and gradually explored in clinical practice. Its effectiveness has been demonstrated in multiple clinical trials. Retroauricular administration can achieve satisfactory drug concentrations in the inner ear while reducing the potential side effects of systemic administration. It also avoids damage to the tympanic membrane and middle ear. It is recommended as a salvage treatment for systemic glucocorticoid administration in the latest domestic guidelines for SSNHL.

Systemic administration, most commonly through oral and intravenous routes, is actually two different administration methods. Oral administration involves absorption through the gastrointestinal tract before entering the bloodstream. It has been discovered that 70% of the body's immune cells are located in the gastrointestinal tract. Oral glucocorticoid administration has an inhibitory effect on the immune function of the intestine. Whether this effect is beneficial or detrimental depends on the specific situation. Additionally, the amount of drug absorbed into the bloodstream through the intestines will always be less than the amount administered directly through intravenous injection. In other words, although both are systemic administration methods, intravenous administration achieves higher concentrations of steroids in the inner ear compared to oral administration. Unilateral SSNHL is often caused by local lesions and is therefore recommended to be treated with intravenous administration. Bilateral SSNHL is primarily influenced by systemic factors, and oral glucocorticoid administration is recommended.

Currently, there are two methods of local administration: intratympanic administration and retroauricular administration. With intratympanic administration, the drug enters the inner ear and primarily distributes in the basal turn and vestibule of the cochlea, including the scala vestibuli and scala tympani, with the highest concentration in the perilymph. The research findings of our team were published as a cover article in *Hearing Research*, indicating that the distribution pattern of hormones in the cochlea differs depending on the administration route. After systemic administration, hormones are distributed more in the vascular stria, while local administration leads to a higher distribution in the Corti organ. Among the three administration routes, intratympanic administration generates higher drug concentrations in the basal turn (high-frequency region), while systemic administration and retroauricular administration achieve higher drug concentrations in the apical turn (low-frequency region). This suggests that the administration route may affect the efficacy of different types of SSNHL. Therefore, different administration methods can be used for different types of lesions. For basal turn and vestibular lesions, such as high-frequency deafness and some vestibular diseases like Tumarkin attacks or dizziness after sound stimulation, intratympanic administration is recommended. For low-frequency sensorineural hearing loss, Ménière's disease, and vestibular migraine, retroauricular administration is expected to be more effective than intratympanic administration. It is worth noting that the advantage of intratympanic administration is that the drug does not enter the bloodstream, but the disadvantage is also that it does not enter the bloodstream. If the lesion is located in the blood vessels of the inner ear, intratympanic administration alone will not be effective. Retroauricular administration allows a portion of the drug to enter the bloodstream, but the concentration in the blood is very low.

Regarding whether local administration can replace systemic administration, in fact, the four administration methods, oral, intravenous, intratympanic, and retroauricular, are not mutually exclusive. They have different mechanisms of action and targets and can be used in combination.

9.6.1.3 Systemic Administration

The first-line treatment for SSNHL is recommended to be systemic administration. Glucocorticoids may exert their effects on the inner ear by inhibiting immune responses, improving microcirculation, and reducing endolymphatic hydrops. Systemically administered drugs enter the inner ear target organ through the bloodstream and exert their effects by binding to glucocorticoid receptors in the inner ear. Additionally, during the process of reaching the target organ, they can directly act on damaged vascular endothelium and the auditory system.

(1) *Drug Selection: Dexamethasone, Methylprednisolone, or Betamethasone*

1) *Dexamethasone:* The commonly used clinical formulation is oral dexamethasone acetate tablets. It is a classic intermediate-acting glucocorticoid with a low price and convenient oral administration, making it widely used in clinical practice. Its advantages include a lower degree of suppression of the hypothalamic-pituitary-adrenal (HPA) axis. However, it has notable drawbacks. Dexamethasone needs to undergo metabolism in the liver to be converted into active prednisolone, which possesses antiinflammatory activity. Therefore, *caution should be exercised when using dexamethasone in patients with liver disease*. Additionally, the concomitant use of other liver-metabolized drugs should be considered, as it may further burden the liver and cause abnormal liver function. Bazuetamase, a first-line medication for SSNHL treatment, is metabolized in the liver and can cause hepatic dysfunction as a side effect. Hence, when used together, monitoring of liver function indicators is necessary. Although dexamethasone exhibits reduced mineralocorticoid activity, it still retains 0.8 of its activity, which can lead to sodium and water retention at high doses. Special attention should be given when used concomitantly with potassium-sparing diuretics (such as thiazide or loop diuretics), as it may result in excessive potassium loss. Patients with concomitant hypertension should be cautious regarding blood pressure regulation. Overall, dexamethasone is more suitable for low-dose long-term use.

2) *Methylprednisolone:* The commonly used clinical formulations are oral methylprednisolone (Medrol) and methylprednisolone sodium succinate injection. As an intermediate-acting glucocorticoid, its main advantage lies in its extremely high affinity for glucocorticoid receptors, being 600 times stronger than dexamethasone. It exerts its antiinflammatory effects directly in the body without requiring liver conversion, and it has a lower degree of suppression of the HPA axis. However, it still retains half of the mineralocorticoid activity, so attention should be paid to the effects of sodium and water retention during medication. Its unit price is higher, which increases the treatment cost for patients. Currently, in the glucocorticoid pulse therapy for SSNHL, methylprednisolone is the recommended systemic medication.

3) *Betamethasone:* The commonly used clinical formulation is betamethasone sodium phosphate injection, which is a long-acting glucocorticoid. Its advantages include strong antiinflammatory effects and high receptor affinity. It exerts its antiinflammatory effects directly in the body without requiring liver conversion and does not cause sodium and water retention. However, its disadvantages include a long duration of action and a prolonged suppression of the HPA axis with high intensity. It has a low price and is more widely used in primary healthcare institutions. Nevertheless, due to its potent antiinflammatory effects, it also carries the highest risk of side effects. When used continuously, attention should be given to the drug's cumulative effect, and the dosage should be adjusted appropriately. Long-term use is not recommended. *The biological half-life of betamethasone is approximately*

Table 9.2 In vivo drug metabolism accumulation of dexamethasone 10 mg × 10 days

Days	1	2	3	4	5	6	7	8	9	10
1	10	7.5	5	2.5	1					
2		10	7.5	5	2.5	1				
3			10	7.5	5	2.5	1			
4				10	7.5	5	2.5	1		
5					10	7.5	5	2.5	1	
6						10	7.5	5	2.5	1
7							10	7.5	5	2.5
8								10	7.5	5
9									10	7.5
10										10
Total volume (mg)	10	17.5	22.5	25	26	26	26	26	26	26

190 min, and the tissue half-life is about 3 days. Accumulation can reach 26 mg on the fifth day (equivalent to approximately 175 mg of dexamethasone) and persist until the tenth day. Please refer to Table 9.2 for more details.

(2) *Dosage and Treatment Duration*

The dosage and treatment duration for glucocorticoid therapy in SSNHL vary across different guidelines. The 2012 American guidelines recommend an oral dose of prednisone at 1 mg/kg/day, with a maximum daily dose of 60 mg. The recommended treatment duration is 10–14 days, emphasizing that the total medication dosage should reach 540 mg. The German guidelines suggest a 5-day course of oral prednisone at 1 mg/kg/day for pulse therapy. The Chinese guidelines for SSNHL, based on a multicenter study conducted in China in 2015, recommend a daily dose of 60 mg of prednisone for 3 days. If effective, the treatment can be extended to 5 days. Alternatively, an equivalent dose of methylprednisolone or dexamethasone can be administered intravenously, with a maximum total dose of 300 mg. These options fall under short-term pulse therapy.

Moreover, the Chinese guidelines for SSNHL recommend the German treatment plan for systemic steroid therapy rather than the high-dose 2-week regimen recommended by the American guidelines. The current viewpoint suggests that SSNHL is mostly caused by acute vascular disorders and requires short-term pulse therapy with steroids, rather than long-term steroid use. The American guidelines are more suitable for conditions involving nerve damage, such as Bell's palsy. Therefore, if the patient is suspected to have cochlear neuritis, the American treatment plan can be considered.

1) *Dosage:* The basic mechanism of glucocorticoids' antiinflammatory effect is their binding to glucocorticoid receptors in the cytoplasm of target cells, which affects the transcription of certain genes involved in inflammation and produces antiinflammatory effects. Taking prednisone as an example, when the dosage is between 0.15 and 0.6 mg/kg or 7.5–30 mg/day, the occupancy rate of glucocorticoid receptors ranges from 50% to 100%. When the dosage is between 0.6 and 2 mg/kg or 30–100 mg/day, the occupancy rate reaches 100%. Therefore, it is estimated that a dosage of 60 mg/day achieves 100% receptor occupancy. A multicenter prospective cohort study showed that the choice between lower-dose methylprednisolone and higher-dose dexamethasone had no impact on the efficacy in patients with sudden sensorineural hearing loss. This may be related to the higher receptor binding affinity of methylprednisolone, where even lower doses can achieve receptor saturation and produce a 100% antiinflammatory effect. This also suggests that the application of glucocorticoids is not "the more, the better." Therefore, the guidelines recommend using methylprednisolone in short-term pulse therapy to reduce the overall glucocorticoid dosage.

2) *Treatment duration:* A treatment duration of less than 5 days is considered pulse therapy, which allows for rapid discontinuation of the medication and has fewer side effects. Prolonged and high-dose administration of glucocorticoids can lead to complications such as endocrine and metabolic disorders, gastrointestinal ulceration, bleeding or perforation, infection exacerbation or induction, electrolyte imbalances, and osteoporosis. Particularly, patients with conditions such as diabetes, hypertension, and gastric ulcers are more susceptible to adverse reactions. Additionally, high-dose glucocorticoid therapy can stimulate bone marrow hematopoiesis, leading to an increase in red blood cells, hemoglobin, platelets, fibrinogen concentration, and a shorter clotting time. It can also stimulate the release of neutrophils from the bone marrow into the bloodstream. Currently, it is believed that the main mechanism of SSNHL is microcirculation disorders in the inner ear caused by various factors. Therefore, it is speculated that long-term high-dose glucocorticoid therapy may increase blood viscosity, worsen microcirculation disorders, and affect the efficacy of hemorheological treatment. Thus, the latest guidelines for SSNHL emphasize combination therapy and recommend early short-term pulse therapy with glucocorticoids in conjunction with hemorheological treatment for better outcomes.
3) *Discontinuation:* Exogenous administration of glucocorticoids can suppress the HPA axis, and rapid discontinuation of glucocorticoids may induce symptoms of adrenal insufficiency. Therefore, if the treatment regimen from the American guidelines is selected (maximum daily dose of 60 mg, treatment duration of 10–14 days, emphasizing a total medication dosage of 540 mg), or if other glucocorticoids are used at high doses for more than 7 days, a gradual tapering of the dosage is necessary before complete discontinuation. Prednisone can be reduced by 5–10 mg/day every 3–5 days. Discontinuing dexamethasone can be more challenging as it accumulates in the body and has a significant impact on the HPA axis. Therefore, long-term use of dexamethasone should be avoided in clinical practice. *There have been cases reported in China where the use of dexamethasone at a dose of 10 mg for 10 consecutive days to treat SSNHL resulted in avascular necrosis of the femoral head and led to medical disputes.*

(3) *Route of Administration: Oral or Intravenous?*

The commonly used routes of administration for systemic glucocorticoids are oral administration of prednisone and methylprednisolone and intravenous infusion of dexamethasone and betamethasone. The American guidelines only mention oral administration of prednisone and do not compare it with intravenous or oral administration of other glucocorticoids. This may be related to the healthcare system in the United States, where intravenous infusion is typically performed by doctors and incurs additional costs of \$50–\$100 per session. To reduce medical expenses, there is a tendency to minimize the use of intravenous infusion in Europe and the United States. Currently, a large-scale clinical study is being conducted in Germany to compare the efficacy of oral and intravenous administration of glucocorticoids. In the guidelines in China, it is recommended to use oral prednisone or intravenous methylprednisolone and dexamethasone at equivalent doses. There is no definitive conclusion regarding the effectiveness and safety of oral versus intravenous administration of glucocorticoids for the treatment of SSNHL, both domestically and internationally. There is a lack of large-scale prospective cohort studies on this topic. However, studies on other diseases have shown that long-term oral administration of glucocorticoids is safer than intravenous administration. Oral administration of glucocorticoids can be absorbed by approximately 80–90% and offers more flexibility in terms of dosing, making it suitable for patients without intravenous access. Intravenous administration results in rapid distribution and onset of action, making it suitable for short-term pulse therapy in SSNHL. If the patient's medical conditions permit, intravenous administration is recommended.

(4) *Timing of Administration*

Endogenous glucocorticoid secretion follows a diurnal rhythm, with peak levels occurring at 8 am and trough levels around midnight. The plasma clearance rate of exogenous glucocorticoids is also influenced by the timing of daily administration. The clearance rate of prednisolone and methylprednisolone is 18–28% lower when administered in the morning compared to nighttime administration. In addition, exogenous glucocorticoids can affect the circadian rhythm of cortisol. To minimize the suppression of the HPA axis and maximize the drug's efficacy, it is recommended to administer glucocorticoids around 8 am once daily.

(5) *Contraindications and Precautions*

Before initiating glucocorticoid therapy, careful consideration should be given to the possible contraindications and potential adverse reactions associated with the selected medication. The assessment of risk factors for adverse reactions in patients should be taken into account as an important reference when determining the safety of glucocorticoid therapy, as well as the choice of drug and dosage. Patients with risk factors such as hypertension, diabetes, peptic ulcers, recent fractures, glaucoma, (chronic) infections, lipid abnormalities, and concurrent use of other medications may experience severe adverse reactions and should consider reducing the dose or avoiding systemic administration altogether.

1) In clinical practice, for well-controlled patients with hypertension, diabetes, and cerebrovascular diseases, it is recommended to monitor blood pressure, blood glucose, and other indicators and provide appropriate supportive treatment. For poorly controlled patients, a reduction in dose or avoidance of systemic administration should be considered. Strong glucocorticoids should be avoided in patients with hypertension.
2) *Peptic ulcer* is one of the side effects of glucocorticoids and is dose-related. As the high-dose regimen for SSNHL entails the use of glucocorticoids at the higher end of the standard dosage range, it is recommended to add proton pump inhibitors (PPIs) or other gastric mucosal protectants. This is particularly important for patients who are concurrently using nonsteroidal antiinflammatory drugs or have a history of gastrointestinal ulcers or a family history of ulcers.
3) According to the results of a multicenter study on SSNHL in China, the average age of onset is 42 years, with 51.95% of patients being female. Therefore, consideration should be given to menopausal women in the high-risk population, and the potential side effect of glucocorticoids causing *osteoporosis* should be taken into account. It is recommended to supplement with calcium and vitamin D during glucocorticoid treatment, and phosphate preparations may be added if necessary.
4) Patients with *glaucoma* should avoid glucocorticoid use. However, drug-induced glaucoma generally occurs with local administration or prolonged systemic use of glucocorticoids. If ocular symptoms occur during treatment, eye pressure should be promptly examined.
5) Additionally, literature suggests that glucocorticoids increase the risk of inducing *psychiatric and neurological symptoms* at doses above 40 mg/day, with a significantly higher risk at doses above 80 mg/day. These symptoms often occur within the first week of treatment and can include increased central excitability, euphoria, agitation, insomnia, mental disturbances, depression, and seizures.
6) The use of glucocorticoids during *pregnancy* is still a subject of debate regarding its impact on fetal development. Generally, it is believed that prednisone has limited placental transfer, and doses below 30 mg/day have minimal effects on

the fetus. Dexamethasone, on the other hand, can pass through the placenta, and even low doses can affect fetal development. Therefore, glucocorticoid use should be cautious during pregnancy, especially in the early stages.

7) The use of physiological or maintenance doses of glucocorticoids in *lactating* women generally has no significant adverse effects on infants. However, if lactating women receive moderate or high doses of glucocorticoids as part of an intermediate treatment regimen, breastfeeding should be avoided to prevent potential adverse effects of glucocorticoids secreted in breast milk on the infant.
8) Glucocorticoids can affect the *growth and development* of children. Long-term use of high-dose steroids (prednisone 1 mg/kg/day) can inhibit growth in children, so caution should be exercised when prescribing glucocorticoids to children, aiming for short duration and low doses.

9.6.1.4 *Local Administration*

Due to the presence of the blood-labyrinth barrier, systemic administration of glucocorticoids makes it difficult for the drugs to reach the inner ear at the required concentration and duration for treatment. Increasing the dosage and prolonging the administration time can enhance the effective dose of the drug in the inner ear but may lead to adverse reactions in other systems of the body. Since half a century ago, scholars have begun exploring the local administration of glucocorticoids. Currently, the more mature methods of local administration are intratympanic administration and postauricular administration.

(1) *Intratympanic Administration*

In intratympanic administration, the drug enters the inner ear through the round window or oval window membrane, thus bypassing the blood-labyrinth barrier and achieving a higher concentration of the drug in the inner ear, resulting in good clinical outcomes. However, intratympanic administration carries potential risks such as tympanic membrane perforation and otitis media, and the drug can be lost through the Eustachian tube, leading to unstable sustained drug delivery. A surgical exploration of over 170 cases of patients with profound sudden sensorineural hearing loss in Germany found that approximately 30% of the patients had the round window blocked by scar tissue or granulation tissue. The commonly used methods of intratympanic administration include tympanic membrane puncture, tympanostomy tube placement, administration via the Eustachian tube, and placement of a minipump on the round window membrane. Commonly used drugs include dexamethasone, betamethasone, and methylprednisolone. The American guidelines consider intratympanic administration and systemic administration as equivalent initial treatment options, while the Chinese guidelines emphasize early combination therapy and intratympanic administration as salvage treatment after unsuccessful systemic glucocorticoid therapy.

1) *Drug Selection*

① *Dexamethasone:* The commonly used clinical formulation is dexamethasone sodium phosphate, which is water-soluble and exerts antiinflammatory effects directly in the body without hepatic conversion. It can penetrate the (oval) window membrane and enter the inner ear.

② *Methylprednisolone:* The commonly used clinical formulation is methylprednisolone sodium succinate injection, which is water-soluble and exerts antiinflammatory effects directly in the body without hepatic conversion. It can penetrate the (oval) window membrane and enter the inner ear. It should be noted that the solvent contains benzyl alcohol, which can cause irritation to the tympanic mucosa during intratympanic injection, resulting in strong pain sensation.

③ Other drugs: Drugs such as ciclesonide and budesonide are newly developed synthetic glucocorticoids with good water solubility and increased lipid solubility, making them more easily absorbed by mucous membranes. Therefore, clinical trials have begun to explore their use in intratympanic administration, but large-scale clinical studies are still lacking.

There is currently no consensus on whether dexamethasone or methylprednisolone is more effective in previous clinical studies on intratympanic administration.

2) *Dosage and Treatment Duration*

Due to the limited volume of the tympanic cavity, the dosage of medication is restricted and generally should not exceed 0.5 mL. Literature shows that higher drug concentrations lead to better efficacy. However, due to the current limitations of clinical drug formulations, the most commonly used formulations are dexamethasone sodium phosphate 5 mg/1 mL and methylprednisolone 40 mg/mL. Therefore, an equal volume of 0.5 mL is administered, with the equivalent dose of methylprednisolone being higher than dexamethasone (3.75:2.5). Additionally, methylprednisolone has a higher glucocorticoid receptor affinity than dexamethasone, suggesting that in clinical practice, the use of methylprednisolone in the tympanic cavity may potentially yield better results.

It is recommended to determine the dosage interval based on the duration of action of different medications. For example, dexamethasone has a duration of action of 36–54 h, so administration every other day is recommended. Methylprednisolone has a duration of action of 12–36 h and can be administered continuously. Based on previous literature, the general number of administrations should not exceed 7 times, and the duration should not exceed 14 days.

3) *Administration Methods*

Tympanic membrane puncture and injection into the tympanic cavity are the most commonly used methods in clinical practice, both domestically and internationally. The advantages of this method include minimal trauma and ease of operation. However, its limitations lie in the inability to accurately control the amount of medication reaching the round window membrane and the duration of contact between the medication and the round window membrane. Tympanic membrane puncture is performed by puncturing the anterior-inferior or posterior-inferior quadrant of the tympanic membrane, and 0.5 mL of dexamethasone or methylprednisolone is injected each time. After sitting for the injection, the patient is instructed to tilt their head 45° toward the opposite side, or if lying down, keep the affected ear facing upward for 30 min, avoiding swallowing and talking as much as possible. During the treatment period, it is important to keep the external auditory canal dry and prevent middle ear infections. In addition to tympanic membrane puncture, other administration methods such as suction tube core administration, microcatheter-controlled administration, and eustachian tube administration are also used. Furthermore, more controlled-release drug delivery devices are under research.

(2) *Postauricular Administration*

Postauricular administration is a minimally invasive administration method that has been recently discovered and gradually studied in clinical practice. Extensive clinical practice has demonstrated the safety and effectiveness of postauricular administration. In animal experiments, postauricular administration under the same dosage has been shown to achieve relatively high concentrations in the inner ear, with a longer duration of action. Furthermore, it maintains relatively low concentrations in the systemic circulation, thereby reducing the potential for systemic side effects caused by glucocorticoids. It is speculated that after postauricular administration, the drug enters the inner ear through various pathways, including systemic circulation, local penetration, and the sigmoid sinus-inner lymphatic sac connection. The main pathway may be through the convergence of drugs via the sigmoid sinus, followed by the close vascular network between the sigmoid sinus and the inner lymphatic sac and then entering the inner lymphatic fluid, thereby directly exerting its effects in the inner ear.

1) *Selection of Medications*

   Currently, commonly used medications for postauricular administration include methylprednisolone, dexamethasone, and betamethasone (compound betamethasone).

   ① *Dexamethasone:* With a molecular weight of 516.41, dexamethasone has good permeability and can enter the inner ear through various possible pathways in the postauricular region. It should be noted that it may still have the potential to cause side effects such as increased blood glucose levels and blood pressure after entering the systemic circulation.

   ② *Methylprednisolone:* With a molecular weight of 496.53, methylprednisolone can enter the inner ear through various possible pathways in the postauricular region. It is particularly important to note that its solvent contains benzyl alcohol, which is poorly absorbed by the human body and may accumulate at the injection site for a long time, potentially causing necrosis of surrounding muscles. Therefore, during injection, it is necessary to ensure that the injection is done subperiosteally. Additionally, it is prohibited to administer methylprednisolone to children.

   ③ *Betamethasone (compound betamethasone):* This is a compound formulation, with each syringe (1 mL) containing 5 mg of betamethasone dipropionate and 2 mg of betamethasone sodium phosphate. Betamethasone sodium phosphate is water-soluble, while betamethasone dipropionate is lipid-soluble. The water-soluble component acts rapidly, similar to dexamethasone sodium phosphate, while the lipid-soluble component is slowly released in tissues, gradually metabolizing and exerting its effects.

2) *Dosage and Duration of Administration*

   Due to the limitations of local tissues, the dosage for postauricular administration generally does not exceed 1 mL. Dexamethasone has a duration of action of 36–54 h, so it is recommended to administer it every other day. Methylprednisolone has a duration of action of 12–36 h. Considering the local absorption capacity in the postauricular region, the local side effects of administering it every other day would be smaller. Continuous administration can also be attempted, but attention should be paid to the condition of the local skin. Alternating with middle ear administration can also be considered. The lipid-soluble component, betamethasone dipropionate, in compound betamethasone is metabolized slowly in tissues, with a drug metabolism time of more than 10 days. Therefore, it is recommended to have at least a 10-day interval between two injections.

3) *Administration Methods*

   Selection of the injection site in the postauricular region: The flat surface of the posterior ear area, at the level of the external auditory meatus, 0.5–1 cm away from the posterior auricular groove, and the surface projection of the temporal bone mastoid air cell area.

   Different injection methods should be selected based on the specific medication being administered. For water-soluble medications such as methylprednisolone and dexamethasone, they should be injected into the subperiosteal layer, which means that the needle is inserted directly to the bone surface and the injection is given between the bone surface and the periosteum. There may be greater resistance and more noticeable pain during this type of injection, so lidocaine can be used in appropriate amounts to alleviate the pain. Water-soluble medications are rapidly absorbed into the bloodstream through local microcirculation. Subperiosteal injection, due to the barrier of the periosteum, can slow down the local absorption rate and increase the amount of medication that permeates locally. As a compound formulation, betamethasone requires intramuscular injection because betamethasone dipropionate is a slow-release component. This allows for gradual release and effectiveness within muscle tissue. The injection depth for betamethasone is the temporal muscle layer. It is important to note that the injection of betamethasone should be at a certain distance from the auricle and the depth should not be too shallow to avoid the side effects of cartilage and skin atrophy. For detailed clinical precautions, please refer to Table 9.3.

When administering medication behind the ear, it is important to note that both dexamethasone and methylprednisolone contain alcohol, which can cause pain upon injection. To alleviate the patient's discomfort, 1 ml of lidocaine can be mixed with the injection, which not only reduces the patient's pain sensation but also facilitates their acceptance of the treatment. Triamcinolone injections, on the other hand, do not typically cause significant pain, although the dosage is relatively lower.

Furthermore, for patients with SSNHL accompanied by systemic conditions such as hypertension, diabetes, uremia, cancer, and pregnant women, doctors should only provide diagnostic and treatment recommendations and engage in discussions with the patients regarding diagnosis and treatment options. The greatest authority of a doctor lies in fully explaining and informing the patient, but the doctor does not have decision-making power. Various possibilities should be communicated to the patient, allowing them to choose the treatment method, including the use of hormones.

In a recent nationwide survey conducted by our department to understand which treatment options patients are willing to accept, we received over 2000 responses. Currently, it appears that medication administered behind the ear may be more readily accepted by patients. More than half of the doctors and medical institutions have adopted this method.

Table 9.3 Comparison of different glucocorticoids

	Methylprednisolone	Dexamethasone	Depo-Prostone	
Ingredients	Methylprednisolone sodium succinate	Dexamethasone sodium phosphate	Betamethasone sodium phosphate	Betamethasone dipropionate
Type	Medium-acting	Long-acting	Long-acting	
Dosage form	Solution	Solution	Solution	
Solubility	Water soluble	Water soluble	Water soluble	Fat soluble
Molecular weight	496.53	516.41	516.41	504.59
Equivalent dose	4	0.75	0.6	
Maintenance time	12–36	36–54	36~54	>10天
Injection location	Subperiosteal	Subperiosteal	Temporal muscle	
Interval	1–2 days	2 days	>10 days	
Side effects	Pain	Pain	Skin atrophy	

9.6.2 Use of Batroxobin

Batroxobin is a purified single-component preparation of refined arginine protease extracted from the venom of Bothrops moojeni, a type of pit viper. It is a thrombin-like enzyme. It can induce the release of tissue plasminogen activator from endothelial cells, decompose fibrinogen, inhibit thrombus formation, and also reduce blood viscosity, inhibit red blood cell aggregation, enhance red blood cell deformability and vascular permeability, reduce vascular resistance, accelerate blood flow velocity, and improve microcirculation in the inner ear.

Research by Li Shuijing et al. showed that the levels of fibrinogen were not significantly correlated with the occurrence of low-frequency descending hearing loss. However, the occurrence of high-frequency descending, flat descending, and total deafness-type sudden hearing loss was associated with high fibrinogen levels at the time of onset. On the other hand, Fang Xuan et al. analyzed the correlation between fibrinogen levels and the therapeutic effect of sudden sensorineural hearing loss with total frequency descending pattern and found that when the fibrinogen level of the patients before treatment was less than 2 g/L or greater than 4 g/L, the therapeutic effect was poor, with an ineffective rate of 50%. On the third day of treatment, the fibrinogen level reached its lowest value, fluctuating between 0.7 and 0.9 g/L, and the therapeutic effect was the best, with a total effective rate of 73.9–83.3%. The fibrinogen level (Fib7) on the seventh day (±1) of treatment had predictive value for the therapeutic effect. The Fib7 level in effective patients was significantly lower than that in the ineffective group. The therapeutic effect was the best when Fib7 was less than 1 g/L, and the higher the Fib7 value, the higher the ineffective rate. Throughout the treatment process, batroxobin has good safety, with no nasal, oral, gastrointestinal bleeding, or systemic bleeding tendency.

9.6.3 Vasodilators

First, it is necessary to differentiate which blood vessels need to be dilated: arteries, veins, or capillaries. For low-frequency SSNHL, as it is believed to be caused by endolymphatic hydrops, the use of high-dose arterial vasodilators is not recommended. Instead, medications that promote venous vasodilation are suggested, such as batroxobin, low-dose ginkgo biloba extract (usually 2–3 tablets), sodium aescinate, oral ginkgo biloba extract, Maitongling, and high-dose nimodipine. For patients with high-frequency SSNHL, which is often associated with vascular spasm and vascular occlusion, a sufficient dose of nimodipine is recommended. The main effects of nimodipine include the following:

(1) Vasodilation: it can dilate coronary and peripheral blood vessels, as well as cerebral blood vessels, increasing cerebral blood flow.
(2) Antithrombotic effect: it can inhibit ADP and collagen-induced platelet aggregation, increase tissue plasminogen activator (tPA), decrease plasminogen activator inhibitor (PAI), and inhibit platelet thrombus formation.

    Additionally, cilostazol is another option. Its main action is to activate intracellular adenylate cyclase as an exogenous prostaglandin E1, leading to a significant increase in cAMP levels in platelets and vascular smooth muscle, resulting in platelet inhibition and vasodilation. Since the cochlear artery lacks smooth muscle, prostaglandins actually act on the vessels one level above. Therefore, it may be more effective in patients with SSNHL attributed to vascular spasm, especially in diabetic patients.

Traditional Chinese medicine also has vasodilating properties. Different herbs have different characteristics. For example, Danshen (*Salvia miltiorrhiza*) and Honghua (*Carthamus tinctorius*) are commonly used, but they have distinct differences. Danshen's main effect is blood activation, but it also has a blood-nourishing effect, which can generate new blood. Therefore, it may be more suitable for SSNHL patients with anemia. Danshen has a cooling nature and is suitable for use during heat-related conditions or when there are signs of infection. On the other hand,

Honghua has a warming nature and is suitable for resolving blood stasis throughout the body, but it does not have a blood-nourishing effect. Furthermore, Earthworm (*Lumbricus*) has anticoagulant, antithrombotic, and vasodilating effects. Its ability to resolve blood stasis is greater than that of Danshen and Honghua, making it more effective in dispersing blood stasis. Therefore, Earthworm may be more suitable for low-frequency and total deafness SSNHL. Understanding the characteristics, mechanisms of action (target sites), and adverse reactions of medications, including traditional Chinese medicine, is helpful in making the correct choice of treatment.

9.6.4 Neurotrophic Agents

Neurotrophic agents commonly used in the treatment of SSNHL include methylcobalamin, mouse nerve growth factor, and ganglioside GM1. Methylcobalamin is widely used in patients with peripheral neuropathy and can promote axonal transport and regeneration, as well as phospholipid synthesis and neuronal myelination. Mouse nerve growth factor has a role in promoting the recovery of injured nerves and can also reduce the incidence of myelin swelling and the number of degenerative fibers in the tibial nerve of animals. Ganglioside GM1 can promote functional repair of the central nervous system by promoting "neuronal remodeling" (including neuronal survival, axonal growth, and synapse formation). This drug also has a protective effect on secondary nerve degeneration after injury, improves cerebral hemodynamic parameters, and reduces postinjury brain edema by improving the activity of cell membrane enzymes and reducing neuronal cell swelling. In clinical practice, neurotrophic agents may be added for SSNHL, especially in patients with suspected cochlear neuritis. It is generally recommended to first improve vascular function and hormone levels before using neurotrophic agents. Mouse nerve growth factor may have a better repairing effect on total deafness, while ganglioside GM1, due to its "neuronal remodeling" effect, may achieve better results when used in combination with batroxobin, particularly for patients with high-frequency damage.

9.6.5 Antioxidants

Commonly used antioxidants in clinical practice include alpha-lipoic acid, edaravone, and butylphthalide. The antioxidant effect of alpha-lipoic acid is often used in the treatment of peripheral neuropathy in diabetes. Edaravone and butylphthalide are both used as neuroprotective agents during the acute phase of cerebral infarction. They work by inhibiting oxidative damage to nerve cells and suppressing neuronal apoptosis. Therefore, for cases of total deafness, early application of these drugs is recommended. However, the clinical application of antioxidants faces challenges as their pharmacological effects are well established, but their clinical efficacy is not significant. There are several reasons for this. Firstly, in animal experiments, often superhigh or even lethal doses are administered, which may be effective for local cell tissues. It is also necessary to consider whether the drugs can pass the blood-labyrinth barrier and reach the cochlear hair cells. Therefore, although antioxidants are considered, overall, their effectiveness is not prominent.

9.6.6 Other Medications

Minshilang (Betahistine Mesilate) can effectively reduce endolymphatic hydrops, but its therapeutic effect is dose-dependent. Studies abroad have found that the best effect in reducing inner ear hydrops is achieved with a dosage of 48 mg three times daily (Tid), while in China, the usual dosage is 6–12 mg Tid, which is far from sufficient. It is recommended to take 12 mg Tid after meals. If the patient does not experience significant gastrointestinal discomfort after 2–3 days, an additional tablet can be added, gradually increasing the dosage to four tablets per dose. This medication has a good safety profile, with no significant side effects reported after oral administration for several years, allowing for long-term use.

9.6.7 Order of Medication Use

In the pharmacological treatment of SSNHL, different medications should be selected based on the specific type of the condition. For example, the dosage of the same medication, such as Jinna Duo, varies in low-frequency and total deafness patients. Additionally, the guidelines for SSNHL suggest that combination therapy is more effective than monotherapy. However, when using combination therapy, the order of medication administration should be considered as it can also affect the treatment outcome. Taking total deafness as an example, the first step is to use batroxobin to improve vascular circulation (clear the pathway). Then, intravenous administration of steroids can reduce vascular endothelial edema (widen the pathway), followed by the use of drugs that improve microcirculation and antioxidants (supplement nutrients). Generally, neurotrophic agents are added only after some recovery of hearing or the presence of auditory perception. If viral infection is suspected, neurotrophic agents should be administered as early as possible.

9.6.8 Treatment of SSNHL in Children

The principles of treatment for children differ significantly from those for adults. Children generally do not experience inner ear ischemia, and the most common causes of SSNHL in children are viral infections and migraines. Vestibular migraine is the leading cause of dizziness in children, and cochlear migraine can also occur. It is crucial to differentiate between the causes during treatment, as the treatment principles for these two causes differ significantly. When selecting medications, if the efficacy is similar, it is advisable to choose medications with fewer side effects.

9.6.9 SSNHL and Migraine

In 2018, Professor Lai Rencong from Taiwan published an article proposing the concept of cochlear migraine. Prior to this, several articles had already suggested that migraine could be a risk factor for SSNHL. Furthermore, a big data study conducted in Taiwan found that individuals with a history of migraine were more likely to experience tinnitus and other cochlear-related disorders. The incidence of cochlear dysfunction in the migraine group was significantly higher than in the nonmigraine group (81.4% vs. 29.4%).

Migraine has multiple mechanisms, including excessive excitability of vascular nerves, abnormal vascular function, and ion channel abnormalities, among others. Under the influence of these various mechanisms, pathological changes occur in the inner ear, leading to endolymphatic hydrops. Of course, immune responses, trauma, inflammation, and other factors can also cause endolymphatic hydrops. SSNHL triggered by migraine is characterized by recurrent attacks, and the hearing profile may vary with each episode. These variations cannot be fully explained by physical damage alone. Most cases exhibit a predominant low-frequency hearing loss, but severe cases can also present with a total deafness pattern. Therefore, it is speculated that migraine-induced SSNHL may not only lead to endolymphatic hydrops but also cause vascular spasm in the inner ear. Aseptic labyrinthitis is also considered one of the possible mechanisms.

The recovery rate of SSNHL caused by migraine is expected to be the highest, with a high rate of spontaneous recovery. The incidence of migraine accompanying different types of hearing loss varies, with a rate of 10% for low-frequency and high-frequency patterns, 20% for rising-flat patterns, 14% for falling-flat patterns, and around 11% for consistent patterns. Therefore, the rising-flat pattern has the highest incidence rate when accompanied by migraine. For total deafness with a predominant low-frequency hearing loss, it is necessary to consider whether it is related to migraine. In cases where all frequencies exhibit a consistent decrease, and the audiogram shows a flat line, considerations should be given to factors such as vascular spasm, thrombosis, hemorrhage, and cochlear neuritis.

10 Summary of Studies on Postauricular Administration

Yixu Wang, Yatong Zhang, and Lisheng Yu

Due to the significant systemic side effects of systemic administration of glucocorticoids, while tympanic administration is an invasive treatment, otologists have been exploring a safe, effective, and simple administration method for many years. Since Yang Xiaoqi and others first used postauricular administration as a remedial treatment for 23 patients with unilateral low-frequency sensorineural hearing loss, postauricular administration has attracted much attention from domestic scholars due to its unique characteristics with minimal invasion, safety, and high efficacy. The site for administration behind the ear is the surface projection of the mastoid sieve area, which is the plane of the external auditory canal behind the ear and 0.5–1.0 cm outside the groove behind the ear. In 2015, the Chinese guidelines for the diagnosis and treatment of sudden deafness recommended postauricular administration as a salvage treatment for systemic administration. The commonly used drugs for administration are 20–40 mg methylprednisolone or 5–10 mg dexamethasone, once every other day, for 4–5 consecutive doses. If the patient has difficulty in follow-up, it is recommended to use 2 mg (1 ml) of compound betamethasone, which can be injected once. The effectiveness of postauricular administration as initial treatment, salvage treatment, or combination therapy has been confirmed by multiple clinical trials. Jing Yuanyuan et al. performed salvage therapy on 45 patients with SSNHL with full frequency decline. The study found that the ear administration group had a significant therapeutic effect compared to the systemic administration group (average hearing threshold increase of 20.01 ± 14.11 dB vs 10.47 ± 8.53 dB, $p = 0.0087$), especially in improving low-frequency hearing. Wang Mingming et al. initially treated 218 SSNHL patients with postauricular administration. The study found that the recovery rate of the postauricular administration group was 30.3%, the significant effective rate was 18.8%, the effective rate was 15.6%, and the total effective rate was 64.7%. The study by Gao Ziwen et al. showed that the effective rate of treating SSNHL with a combination of postauricular administration and systemic administration was 50%, with an average hearing improvement value of 17.78 ± 18.12 dB.

Y. Wang · Y. Zhang · L. Yu (✉)
Department of Otorhinolaryngology, Head and Neck Surgery, People's Hospital, Peking University, Beijing, China

L. Yu (ed.), *Progress in Postauricular Administration*, Experts' Perspectives on Medical Advances,
https://doi.org/10.1007/978-981-95-5102-6_10

10.1 The Efficacy of Postauricular Administration for the Treatment of Low-Frequency Descending SSNHL

Yang Xiaoqi et al. first reported the effectiveness of using postauricular administration of betamethasone to treat refractory low-frequency declining SSNHL. By treating 23 and 18 cases of low-frequency SSNHL with initial treatment failure with postauricular administration and systemic administration, respectively, it was found that the efficacy of the postauricular administration group was significantly higher than that of the systemic administration group (effective rate 82.6% vs 22.2%, $p < 0.05$); postauricular administration of steroids can effectively treat refractory low-frequency declining SSNHL, but the efficacy is poor for bilateral patients. Wang Mingming et al. compared the efficacy of postauricular administration and systemic administration in the treatment of low to mid frequency SSNHL and found that the recovery rate of the postauricular administration group (65.0%) was significantly higher than that of the systemic administration group (41.7%), with statistical significance ($p < 0.05$), further indicating that postauricular administration of glucocorticoids has the best efficacy in the treatment of low to mid frequency SSNHL. It recommends that postauricular administration is suitable for the treatment of low-frequency descending SSNHL.

10.2 The Efficacy of Postauricular Administration for the Treatment of High-Frequency Descending SSNHL

Wang Mingming et al. compared the efficacy of systemic administration and postauricular administration for the treatment of high-frequency SSNHL and found that the total effective rate of the postauricular administration group was 63.2%, while the total effective rate of the systemic administration group was 75%, while the difference was not statistically significant. But for those with poor blood pressure and blood sugar control, the treatment method of postauricular administration should be chosen. Wang Fei et al. compared the therapeutic effects of systemic and postauricular administration of glucocorticoids for the treatment of high-frequency declining SSNHL and found that the total effective rate of the postauricular administration group was 76.0% while the total effective rate of the systemic administration group was 55.6%. The therapeutic effect of postauricular administration was significant, and the difference was statistically significant.

10.3 The Efficacy of Postauricular Administration for Treating SSNHL with Full Frequency Decline

Zhao Qun et al. explored the efficacy of postauricular administration in the treatment of total deafness SSNHL and found that compared with the systemic administration group, the hearing improvement in the low-frequency range (125–500 Hz) was significantly higher in postauricular administration group, and the difference was statistically significant. In the early stage, our group performed postauricular administration as salvage treatment on 45 cases of total deafness SSNHL. It was found that the group receiving postauricular administration had an increase in the average hearing threshold at all frequencies compared to the group receiving systemic treatment, especially in the low-frequency region (250 Hz, 500 Hz) where the increase was more significant ($p = 0.0018$, $p = 0.0027$). It recommended that postauricular administration has a significant therapeutic effect on SSNHL with full frequency decline, especially in improving low-frequency hearing.

10.4 The Efficacy of Postauricular Administration for Treating Flat SSNHL

Zhao Qun et al. compared the efficacy of postauricular administration and systemic administration for the treatment of flat SSNHL and found that the recovery rate of the postauricular administration group was 24.2%, while the systemic administration group was only 6.7%, with statistical significance. This suggests that postauricular administration can improve the recovery rate of flat SSNHL. However, the study by Wang Mingming et al. showed that the total effective rate of postauricular administration for treating flat SSNHL was 41.2%, while the total effective rate of systemic administration was 32.9%. Although the efficacy of postauricular administration group was higher than the systemic administration group, there was no statistical significance.

10.5 Basic Research on Postauricular Administration

Although large clinical trials have confirmed the efficacy and safety of postauricular administration, basic experiments on postauricular administration are relatively insufficient. The study by Jing Yuanyuan et al. showed that the peak drug concentration in the sigmoid sinus blood of postauricular administration group was 3.03 times higher than that of the systemic administration group, and the area under the sigmoid sinus drug concentration curve was 2.93 times higher than that of the systemic administration group. Postauricular administration can maintain high drug concentration in the sigmoid sinus and lower drug concentration in the systemic circulation. Postauricular administration can maintain a high local drug concentration while reducing the possibility of systemic side effects caused by glucocorticoids. Lin Yunjuan et al. used enzyme-linked immunosorbent assay to measure and compare the drug concentrations in the inner ear between postauricular administration and systemic administration. They found that postauricular administration had higher local drug concentrations in the inner ear than systemic administration, and the difference was statistically significant ($p < 0.05$), with unique characteristics such as earlier peak time and longer duration. Li et al. used 7.0T MRI to measure and compare the signal time curves of systemic administration and postauricular administration. They found that compared with systemic administration, postauricular administration has the characteristics of a larger area under the drug curve, a later peak time, and a larger total amount of drugs acting on the inner ear. Shi Jiao et al. compared the concentration time curves of perilymphatic drugs between postauricular administration and intratympanic administration and found that although the concentration of perilymphatic drugs in postauricular administration was significantly lower than that in intratympanic administration, it had the characteristics of long half-life period and early peak time. Chen Aiping et al. used visible light imaging technology in animals to study the action pathway and pharmacokinetic characteristics of postauricular administration. They found that postauricular administration has a significant sustained release effect, can maintain a relatively long drug concentration locally, and has less distribution in other organs throughout the body. Diao Tongxiang et al. used fluorescein isothiocyanate dextran (FITC Dextran) as a tracer to explore the possible pathway of postauricular administration. They found that drugs are more likely to enter the endolymphatic fluid in postauricular administration than systemic administration. It is speculated that the tracer reaches the sigmoid sinus and then enters the endolymphatic fluid through the choroidal connection between the sigmoid sinus and the endolymphatic sac. Wang et al. found that the distribution characteristics of steroids in the cochlea vary through different routes of administration. After systemic administration, steroids are more distributed in the vascular lines, while local administration is more distributed in the Corti apparatus. Among the three routes of administration, intratympanic administration produces higher drug concentrations in the cochlear floor (high-frequency region), while systemic administration and postauricular administration have higher drug concentrations in the cochlear top (low-frequency region) than tympanic administration, suggesting that the administration route may affect in different types of sudden deafness. Therefore, different types of lesions can be treated with different administration methods.

In summary, postauricular administration can produce higher concentrations of drugs in the inner ear and sigmoid sinus blood compared to systemic administration, while maintaining lower systemic drug concentrations and longer duration of drugs in the inner ear. Compared with intratympanic administration, although the concentration of perilymphatic drugs is lower, they have the characteristics of longer half-life and earlier peak time. The postauricular administration of glucocorticoid not only has little impact on the blood pressure and blood sugar of the whole body but also is suitable for patients with diabetes and hypertension and can effectively avoid the disadvantages of invasive tympanic administration and drug instability [1].

10.6 Possible Pathways of Action for Postauricular Administration

At present, it is believed that drugs may reach the inner ear through multiple pathways such as systemic circulation, anatomical fissure infiltration, and sigmoid sinus endolymphatic sac after being injected into the postauricular area.

10.6.1 Systemic Circulation Pathway

After injection through the ear, some drugs may enter the systemic circulation through two pathways. (1) The drug is first absorbed through the capillaries and lymphatic vessels behind the ear and then flows into the external jugular vein through the postauricular vein and finally enters the systemic circulation through the subclavian vein. (2) The drug enters the sigmoid sinus directly through the mastoid vein and then flows back into the systemic circulation through the internal jugular vein. The drug then enters the skull through the internal carotid artery and vertebral artery system and finally divides into the vestibular artery and cochlear artery through the labyrinthine artery to reach the inner ear.

10.6.2 Anatomical Fracture Infiltration Pathways

In the anatomy of the temporal bone in normal individuals, some natural fissures such as the tympanic fissure and the ethmoid area exist behind the ear and middle ear. These natural fissures communicate with each other, allowing small molecule substances such as dexamethasone to enter the middle ear through permeation from the behind ear area. Cros et al. used micro CT technology to measure the temporal bone of humans and found a large number of tiny channels connecting the middle ear and mastoid process. After medication is administered through the ear, it may enter the middle ear directly through a small channel. The medication that enters the middle ear then passes through the circular window membrane or stapes area and enters the inner ear.

10.6.3 Sigmoid Sinus Endolymphatic Sac Pathway

After injection through the ear, the drug is absorbed into the bloodstream by local capillaries or lymphatic vessels, flows into the ear vein, and then partially enters the systemic circulation through the external jugular vein into the subclavian vein. The other part reaches the sigmoid sinus directly through the mastoid vein. The sigmoid sinus is located at the distal end of the endolymphatic sac, and the two are tightly connected through connective tissue. The lymphatic sac is surrounded by a vascular network formed by capillaries, lymphatic capillaries, venules, and arterioles, which flow back to the sigmoid sinus through the vestibular aqueduct vein. The drug may be injected behind the ear and spread to the internal lymphatic sac after reaching the sigmoid sinus. Drugs in the sigmoid sinus may enter the endolymphatic sac through the choroidal connection between the sigmoid sinus and the endolymphatic sac. Friis and Qvortrup blocked the distal end of the vestibular aqueduct in experimental animals, observed the vestibular vein under a fluorescence microscope, and found reverse blood flow to the inner ear, thus inferring that venous blood from the sigmoid sinus can flow back into the inner ear.

Reference

1. Wang Y, Han L, Diao T, et al. A comparison of systemic and local dexamethasone administration: From perilymph/cochlea concentration to cochlear distribution [J]. Hear Res. 2018;370:1–10.

Mechanisms of Subjective Tinnitus 11

Xin Ma, Yuting Tao, and Lisheng Yu

11.1 Introduction

Tinnitus is one of the most common and refractory disorders [1, 2]. The term is derived from the Latin word "tinnire" which meaning to ring. Tinnitus is a common occurrence that nearly everyone has encountered at least once in their lifetime. Typically, it vanishes within a short period of time, ranging from seconds to hours. Nevertheless, enduring tinnitus can have an impact on mental well-being and social functioning [3].

Tinnitus can be categorized into two distinct categories. Objective tinnitus refers to the presence of genuine physical sound wave vibrations that can be perceived by others or recorded using instruments, such as pulsatile tinnitus [4]. Subjective tinnitus, on the other hand, describes the sensation of meaningless sounds in the absence of external sound sources. Majorly, patients complaining of tinnitus are experiencing subjective tinnitus, while its mechanism remains elusive. This chapter demonstrates the integrated regulation theory of subjective tinnitus and pathogenetic factors of subjective tinnitus.

11.2 Pathophysiology

11.2.1 Hearing Loss and Tinnitus

The majority of individuals with tinnitus display measurable hearing loss [5]. However, they sometimes cannot feel the loss of hearing themselves, especially when it progresses gradually. Studies have revealed the correlation between the frequency of tinnitus and the region of hearing loss in the audiogram. For patients with sudden hearing losses such as sudden sensorineural hearing loss (SSNHL) or noise-induced hearing loss (NIHL), tinnitus commonly occurs as a concomitant symptom. Additionally, outer hair cell dysfunction has been revealed among individuals with tinnitus. Consequently, tinnitus has long been seen as predominantly caused by inner ear diseases. However, among 414 patients with acoustic neuromas who experienced auditory nerve sectioning, only 40% reported relief of tinnitus, which was equivalent to placebo effects. Additionally, many patients reporting hearing loss do not suffer from tinnitus, while some with normal hearing may have tinnitus. These observations show that hearing loss is not the only factor accounting for the development of tinnitus.

X. Ma · Y. Tao · L. Yu (✉)
Department of Otorhinolaryngology, Head and Neck Surgery, People's Hospital, Peking University, Beijing, China
e-mail: 1810301239@pku.edu.cn

L. Yu (ed.), *Progress in Postauricular Administration*, Experts' Perspectives on Medical Advances,
https://doi.org/10.1007/978-981-95-5102-6_11

11.2.2 Neurophysiological Models of Tinnitus

One innovative step of understanding the mechanism of tinnitus is recognizing the role of the central nervous system (CNS). J. Tonndorf was one of the initial researchers to correlate tinnitus development with the CNS. Jastreboff originally developed a neurophysiological model of tinnitus, positing that peripheral hearing loss serves merely as a triggering factor for tinnitus, while subsequent rearrangement of central auditory pathways is the major cause of tinnitus [2]. This paradigm considers tinnitus as a central nervous remodeling disorder, while negative emotions toward tinnitus generated by limbic system lead to chronicization of tinnitus. This neurophysiological model of tinnitus and treatments evolved from it have held major significance in this field.

11.2.3 Neural Remodeling Within the Auditory System

It has been proven that mature auditory system retains the plasticity and can adapt itself to respond to any modifications in the auditory environment. Numerous factors, including auditory deprivation, excessive sound stimulation, and endogenous inflammation, might stimulate neuroplasticity to compensate for hearing loss, ultimately resulting in the development of tinnitus.

11.2.3.1 Excitation-Inhibition Imbalance

Auditory signals can simultaneously trigger both excitatory and inhibitory responses in the same auditory nerve fiber. Following hearing loss, there is an imbalance between excitatory and inhibitory responses in nerve fibers, leading to hyperexcitability of the auditory nerve, which may result in tinnitus.

11.2.3.2 Lateral Inhibition

When a neuron is stimulated and then causes its nearby neuron to become activated, the latter might suppress the excitatory response of the former. This condition is particularly common in the thalamus. An increase in the rate of spike is spotted in particular neurons in the thalamus in hearing-impaired individuals, suggesting hyperexcitability in the ascending auditory pathway due to auditory deprivation. These electrical signals may be experienced as tinnitus.

11.2.3.3 Neural Synchronization

In animals with normal hearing, neurons exhibit specificity in acoustic frequency, and the auditory cortex is also structured spatially according to their correlating frequency. Hearing loss results in disruption of the primary auditory cortex, with neurons in damaged parts of the auditory cortex moving their frequency preference toward the surrounding frequency. Enhanced electric activity around the damaged region may constitute the basis for tinnitus development. However, tinnitus frequencies generally match the impaired regions rather than the proximate area, suggesting that neuronal synchronization at the deteriorated site may contribute to tinnitus.

11.2.3.4 Impaired Function of the Auditory Descending System

When the contralateral ear receives auditory stimulation, the medial olivocochlear bundle crossing over to the contralateral outer hair cells releases the neurotransmitter acetylcholine to hyperpolarize the membrane potential and inhibit the active movement of outer hair cells. Once hearing function is impaired, the efferent function of the medial olivocochlear bundle decreases, stimulating outer hair cell function and increasing the afferent efficiency of the auditory system. Studies have shown that 90% of patients with tinnitus exhibit inner ear dysfunction, especially outer hair cell dysfunction, and approximately 50% of patients with tinnitus and hyperacusis reveal enhanced outer hair cell function, which may be related to the decreased efferent neural function from the medial olivocochlear bundle.

11.2.4 Neuroplasticity Outside the Auditory System

The ascending auditory pathway contains both classical and nonclassical mechanisms. In the classical pathway, neurons in the thalamic nuclei project progressively to the primary and secondary auditory cortices. However, in the nonclassical pathway, projections bypass the primary cortex and directly target the secondary auditory cortex. Apart from the auditory system, the nonclassical pathway can accept inputs from other systems, such as the somatosensory and visual systems. It has been confirmed that there are exact connections between the trigeminal nucleus and the dorsal cochlear nucleus, as well as between the upper spinal cord and the dorsal cochlear nucleus. Input information from different systems is integrated in the dorsal cochlear nucleus. Notably, only in children and patients with tinnitus is the nonclassical pathway activated. After hearing deprivation, neural remodeling affects synaptic efficiency and opens pathways that are ordinarily closed due to inefficient synapses, correcting for diminished auditory input but potentially leading to tinnitus. Activation of the nonclassical pathway can explain the somatic modulation of tinnitus in clinical settings. For instance, treating temporomandibular joint disorders helps alleviate tinnitus in some patients.

11.3 The Emotional System

Approximately 17–30 ms after auditory stimulation, the primary auditory cortex is activated and maintains activated status until 300 ms poststimulation, suggesting parallel pathways within CNS may exist and simultaneously transmit signals to insular cortex or other regions responsible for emotional processing. Both classical and nonclassical pathways involved in auditory compensation are associated with the lateral nucleus of the amygdala. The connection between the classical pathway and the emotional system serves as a high pathway, and its activation is related to the warning role of sounds in survival. The auditory system is always searching for meaningful or possibly threatening sounds in the surrounding environment and adapts itself to irrelevant or harmless sounds. However, the connection between the nonclassical system and the emotional system serves as a low channel and is only observed to be active in children and patients with tinnitus. Researches have demonstrated that activation of the low pathway is more likely to lead to excessive responses from the emotional system compared to the high pathway. Jastreboff supposes that the commencement of the negative emotional system after the development of tinnitus is an essential reason for the chronicization of tinnitus. If patients continue to focus on tinnitus and attribute negative meanings to it, such as tinnitus may worsen over time, tinnitus will lead to deafness, or tinnitus heralds the onset of severe diseases, they will further experience negative emotions amplifying their perception of tinnitus. Controlling these unpleasant and inappropriate psychological responses is key to the therapy of tinnitus.

In summary, according to the neurophysiological model of tinnitus, hearing loss initiates neural remodeling which generates excessive electrical signals within the CNS and results in tinnitus. Additionally, the auditory system is extensively linked to the emotional and somatic systems, contributing to the chronicization of tinnitus. However, this theory is not always consistent with clinical and experimental findings. Animals with temporary threshold shifts following noise exposure can exhibit persistent impairment of the auditory nerve even after complete recovery of hearing, which means neural remodeling continues to occur. However, patients exposed to noise with temporary threshold shifts usually report hearing amelioration with eradication of tinnitus. These findings imply that not all excessive electrical signals generated during neural remodeling are turned into tinnitus. Subsequent researches have demonstrated the participation of tinnitus control systems.

11.4 Integrated Regulation Theory of Tinnitus

The integrated regulation theory of tinnitus introduces a new idea of tinnitus control system. According to this view, at the outset of inner ear injury, hearing loss prompts the brain to become aware and instantly stimulates compensation by the auditory center. Signals that have been transmitted may be perceived as tinnitus. Whether the tinnitus signal can be conveyed depends on the ability of the tinnitus control system. The system includes the gate-control system and the ventilation system.

11.5 The Gate-Control System: Frontal-Striatal Circuit

Hallam et al. hypothesized in 1984 that the brain selectively attends to or ignores specific stimuli for effectiveness. Tinnitus is considered a neutral stimulus for most individuals, and repeated exposure to tinnitus signals gradually leads the CNS to perceive tinnitus as a nonthreatening signal, thus reducing the brain's response to it and gradually diminishing the perception, which is one of the mechanisms of tinnitus self-resolution. This notion is known as the habituation theory of tinnitus and has long remained theoretical without corroborating experimental studies.

Recent studies have shown that the most active auditory compensation after hearing loss occurs at the thalamic level. However, only when electrical signals generated in the primary auditory cortex are processed to auditory cortical network, including the frontal lobe, parietal lobe, and reticular structures can they be sent to the central auditory brain and perceived as tinnitus. Rauschecker JP postulated that these broad network structures operate as gatekeepers, and they are responsible for analyzing and determining whether to transmit these electrical impulses. This intricate network structure may be the site of the tinnitus clearance in CNS.

The degree and speed of hearing loss determine different demands for the central tinnitus clearance system, leading to a complex correlation between tinnitus and hearing loss. The demand for the clearance system and the occurrence of tinnitus increase with the speed and severity of hearing loss, which is compatible with clinical observations. The incidence of tinnitus is particularly high among patients with acute hearing loss, with 90% of SSNHL patients experiencing varied degrees of tinnitus. However, the frequency of tinnitus in people with steady hearing loss is rather low. A study exploring the occurrence of tinnitus in 150 seniors aged 60 and above found that among 78% of participants with hearing loss, 77 had tinnitus at the time of the survey (51.3%) and 35 of them had persistent tinnitus (23.3%), with only 31 cases (20.7%) lasting more than 3 months [6].

11.6 The Ventilation System: Eustachian Tube

Sounds produced by respiration, blood flow, joint movements, and so on are all muted so that they are not recognized by the auditory central nervous system. Researches have demonstrated that the active closure of the eustachian tube in concave-eared frogs induces a attenuation of 26 dB in low-frequency sounds (3–10 kHz) and a boost of 20 dB in high-frequency sounds (10–32 kHz) to highlight ultrasonic signals for communication. The eustachian tube function differs between humans and concave-eared frogs. In human beings, the eustachian tube is funnel-shaped, narrowing from the outside to the interior, with mucosal folds resembling mufflers, allowing the absorption and buffering of sound waves or noise. Some tinnitus signals may be released through the eustachian tube. With eustachian tube dysfunction, tinnitus signals and some normal electrical impulses in the brain cannot be released regularly and may be amplified, making them more likely to be detected, leading to tinnitus.

The integrated regulation theory proposes that tinnitus creation is a complicated process including the central gate control system, the eustachian tube clearance system, the emotional system, and other nonauditory systems throughout the body.

It is revolutionary to recognize the role of nonauditory systems in pathogenesis of tinnitus. Tinnitus is a sensation similar to pain. Just as pain stimuli can induce pain only when they accumulate and reach a particular level, tinnitus is generated when multiple components interact and reach the threshold for tinnitus. It is vital to describe the characteristics of patients dominated by different causes and define classifications and treatments for tinnitus of diverse etiologies.

11.7 Risk Factors

11.7.1 Classifications of Hearing Loss

11.7.1.1 Acute Hearing Loss

In patients with SSNHL, the sudden reduction in auditory input stimulates immediate auditory compensation, resulting in tinnitus as a byproduct of excessive neural activation. Although tinnitus is a distorted sound signal, it can partially compensate for the diminished sound input at the early stage. Therefore, the tinnitus gate control system allows for maximal sound signals and moderate tinnitus signals. Clinical studies have revealed that the severity of tinnitus is not correlated with the degree of hearing loss at the early stage, and tinnitus is generally modest without producing undue anxiety or stress. As the disease stabilizes, tinnitus may lead to unfavorable emotional reactions. However, as the body gradually adapts to hearing loss, the tinnitus control system reactivates and clears the tinnitus signals, resulting in gradual remission of tinnitus.

11.7.1.2 Fluctuating Hearing Loss

Tinnitus induced by fluctuating hearing loss (such as Meniere's disease) can be seen as recurrent bouts of tinnitus due to acute hearing loss, with each episode prompting the presence and clearance of tinnitus. However, once hearing is stabilized, it takes time for tinnitus control system to work. Researches have revealed that most tinnitus can ameliorate over a year. However, if there is not enough time for the control system, tinnitus may progressively accumulate and develop. Therefore, for tinnitus caused by fluctuating hearing loss, treating the primary disease is of great significance.

11.7.1.3 Mild Stable Hearing Loss

Patients with mild stable hearing loss often have hearing loss in the high-frequency range, which may be connected to genetics, age, and persistent noise exposure. Only the minority of patients develop chronic persistent tinnitus. The tinnitus signals created by modest hearing loss are relatively feeble. If the control system works regularly, it can entirely eliminate this level of tinnitus. The occurrence of tinnitus in these patients often implies dysfunction of the tinnitus control system. Therefore, focusing on treating modest irreversible injuries of the ear is not meaningful. Instead, efforts should be made to detect and treat problems that may impact the gate control system and eustachian tube.

11.7.1.4 Moderate to Severe Stable Hearing Loss

As hearing loss gradually worsens, auditory compensation becomes more pronounced, and tinnitus signals accumulate, resulting in persistent tinnitus. Due to age-related changes in central gate control system function, the chance of tinnitus chronicization increases dramatically in the elderly people.

11.7.1.5 Tinnitus with Normal Audiometric Results

Studies have indicated that the proportion of tinnitus patients with normal hearing ranges from 7.4% to 20%, depending on the hearing criteria utilized [5]. In conventional audiometry encompassing the range of 250 Hz–8 kHz, if $\leq$20 dB HL is considered normal, 8% of tinnitus patients have normal hearing. If $\leq$25 dB HL is chosen as the criteria, around 30% of tinnitus patients have normal hearing. In addition, the human ear can receive sound of frequencies from 20 Hz to 20 kHz, which is obviously beyond the range of standard audiometry. Investigations have indicated people with normal hearing in standard audiometric measurements may have abnormalities in extra high frequencies, indicating potential cochlear injury. Auditory brainstem response

(ABR) shows a decrease in the amplitude of the I wave, with normal amplitude of the V wave, indicating that these patients may have hidden hearing loss generating atypical brainstem responses. As a result, routine audiograms may not reveal specific types and degrees of auditory system impairment. Compared to control group, tinnitus patients with normal hearing are likely to have cochlear dead zones or outer hair cell destruction. Animal experiments revealed normal thresholds even when the proportion of damaged outer hair cells has reached 20%. Additionally, animals with normal hearing following noise exposure also reveal subclinical hearing loss. This subclinical or hidden hearing loss may also stimulate aberrant electrical signals in the CNS. However, these electrical impulses are mild and can be eliminated by the tinnitus control system if the system functions regularly, rendering them unnoticeable. Therefore, in the population with hidden hearing loss, tinnitus control system dysfunction is the direct cause of tinnitus, and modifying the control system matters in the treatment of tinnitus.

11.7.2 Physiological Factors

11.7.2.1 Age

It is widely acknowledged that the incidence of tinnitus increases with age, as it in the elderly ranges from 20% to 31.4% in the literature [7–10]. Generally, the central auditory system exhibits both excitatory and inhibitory responses to auditory information. With aging, the inhibitory function weakens, leading to an increase in excessively stimulated tinnitus signals. Additionally, loss in central nervous system function as aging can also reduce the central capacity to filter tinnitus.

11.7.2.2 Insomnia

Secondary insomnia in tinnitus sufferers may be a sign of emotional system malfunction, while primary insomnia may cause tinnitus by altering CNS metabolism. The CNS is the most metabolically active organ in the body. Due to the sensitivity of neurons and glial cells to changes in the extracellular environment, the normal functioning of CNS requires support from lymphatic circulation. Recent researches have confirmed that the perivascular space, located around blood vessels in the brain, functions similarly to the peripheral lymphatic system. The inner wall of the perivascular space is composed of the surfaces of vascular cells, primarily endothelial cells and smooth muscle cells. The outer wall is formed by branches extended from astrocytes unique to the brain and spinal cord. These astrocytes abundantly express aquaporin water channels, facilitating the flow of cerebrospinal fluid. As this system is primarily composed of glial cells, it is known as the glymphatic system. Studies indicate that cerebrospinal fluid is pumped into the brain through channels surrounding arteries, providing comprehensive cleansing, and subsequently drained out through channels surrounding veins. During sleep or under anesthesia, the volume of the interstitial space in brain is 1.6 times that of the awake state, greatly enhancing the function of the glymphatic system. Therefore, sleep plays a crucial role in maintaining metabolic homeostasis within the body. In patients with insomnia, the elimination of metabolic waste by glymphatic system is disturbed, impairing brain function.

11.7.2.3 Migraine

Studies have found that 27% of tinnitus patients experience symptoms of headaches, and there is a significant correlation between the side of the headache and the side of the tinnitus. The current research suggests that the incidence of cochlear abnormalities in migraine and nonmigraine patients is 81.4% and 29.4%, respectively, with a hazard ratio of 2.81 (adjusted to 2.71). Therefore, the concept of cochlear migraine has been postulated as a plausible explanation for persistent tinnitus and recurrent SSNHL. Migraine may affect the development of tinnitus through many processes. Firstly, activated trigeminal nervous system enhances the spontaneous discharge rate of cochlear dorsal nuclei via a crossover pattern. Secondly, the trigeminal nerve innervates the inner ear labyrinth arteries through the ophthalmic branch, and abnormally activated trigeminal axons release neurotransmitters such as calcitonin gene-related peptide (CGRP) and substance P, resulting in inner ear vasodilation, plasma protein extravasation, tissue edema, and a series of sterile inflammatory reactions, thereby initiating or exacerbating tinnitus. Thirdly, migraine with central cortical hypersensitivity substantially inhibits the brain's ability to compensate for tinnitus. Fourthly, many migraine sufferers have comorbidities that affect the development of tinnitus, such as anxiety, depression, hormone imbalances, and insomnia. Among patients with migraine, the prevalence of anxiety and depression is 2–10 times higher than that in the general population, and psychological comorbidity is a significant contributing factor to the chronicization of migraines. In patients with tinnitus accompanying migraine, higher scores on tinnitus handicap inventory are observed, along with lower life quality. Additionally, there is a higher incidence of associated symptoms such as auditory hypersensitivity, vertigo, neck pain, temporomandibular joint disorders, general pain, and depressive symptoms. Furthermore, as a primary brain disorder, migraine may present with many symptoms beyond those specified by the International Headache Society (IHS) criteria. These symptoms include sensitivity to motion, light, odors, pain, and sound, as well as family history of migraine, Meniere's disease or motion sickness, recurrent hearing loss, irritable bowel syndrome, and allergic rhinitis. D. Buchholz noted in *Heal Your Headache* that migraines could trigger any conceivable discomfort in any part of the head or neck. Although these symptoms are currently underrecognized, non-IHS migraine serves as a valuable supplement to migraine diagnosis.

11.7.2.4 Postmenopausal Estrogen Reduction

The development in medicine and technology, coupled with advancement in quality of life, has led to a considerable improvement in human lifespan. The average life expectancy of women in China has reached 75.9 years, with one-third of this time spent after menopause. As ovarian function declines after menopause, resulting to degenerative changes in the body due to the reduction in estrogen levels. Numerous investigations have revealed that the effects of estrogen are far beyond reproductivity. By regulating the growth and development of neurons and synaptic plasticity, estrogen can influence the production and reuptake of neurotransmitters (such as serotonin), alter neuronal excitability, and engage in the regulation of CNS. The decrease in estrogen levels after menopause affects the function of inner ear estrogen receptors, central serotonin neurons, and sympathetic nervous function, thereby affecting the function of the inner ear and the gate control system of tinnitus, leading to the occurrence of weak tinnitus signals that were originally controlled. Due to the relatively low awareness of menopause among the Chinese population and the low incidence of hot flashes among Chinese women, many Chinese menopausal women pay more attention to other symptoms such as tinnitus or paraesthesia pharynges. Otolaryngologists should have an overall medical perspective, carefully exclude other factors related to tinnitus, and select patients whose tinnitus is primarily related to menopausal factors for menopausal therapy.

11.7.2.5 Obstructive Sleep Apnea Hypopnea Syndrome (OSAHS)

Although OSAHS does raise the risk of tinnitus, studies have indicated that only 10–20% of OSAHS patients have experienced tinnitus, and the presence of tinnitus is not correlated to the degree of apnea, suggesting that OSAHS might not be the major risk factor for tinnitus. Some hypothesized that hypoxemia generated by OSAHS may impair auditory function. Furthermore, elevated sympathetic nerve activity and inflammatory responses associated with OSAHS may have a role in the development of tinnitus. Additionally, OSAHS may cause anxiety and depression, further exacerbating tinnitus. Moreover, due to negative intrapleural pressure, OSAHS patients are prone to pharyngoesophageal reflux, which affects the function of the Eustachian tube and middle ear. Furthermore, OSAHS patients have trouble entering deep sleep, resulting in insufficient clearance of metabolic waste in the brain. Also, individuals with OSAHS often have nocturia, diabetes, hypertension, etc., which also have a role in the development of tinnitus.

11.7.2.6 Eustachian Tube System

Common factors that may impact the Eustachian tube system include disorders of the nasal cavity and paranasal sinuses, laryngopharyngeal reflux, and OSAHS. Here we will focus on the impact of laryngopharyngeal reflux on the Eustachian tube and tinnitus. Severe laryngopharyngeal reflux can create otitis media with effusion, in which case tinnitus is merely one of the symptoms rather than a chronic disease. However, many patients do not reveal signs or experimental evidence of otitis media with effusion yet still experience discomfort such as tinnitus and aural fullness. These patients used to be diagnosed with idiopathic tinnitus. They feel changes in tone and clarity when listening to others or self-speaking and usually report the exacerbation of aural fullness when swallowing or speaking. Counterintuitively, aural fullness is commonly ameliorated when lying down. At this time, gastric acid reflux mostly affects the esophagus rather than laryngopharynx and the eustachian tube. Consequently, symptoms are aggravated in the sitting or standing position due to major laryngopharyngeal reflux. Moreover, symptoms are usually minor in the morning and intensify in the evening. It is currently supposed that gastric acid reflux may impact Eustachian tube function by affecting Eustachian tube surfactant. Microscopic examinations reveal that the fold of the Eustachian tube top is predominantly formed by nonciliated cells which can release surfactants similar to pulmonary surfactants composed of phospholipids, polysaccharides, and proteins. Due to the siphon effect, gastric acid expelled into the nasopharynx may be aspirated into the Eustachian tube, potentially impairing the surfactant of the nasopharynx and Eustachian tube, compromising the Eustachian tube opening function. If the acid enters the Eustachian tube and middle ear, it mostly affects the epitympanum, causing mucosal edema around the head of malleus, impairing the motion of the ossicular chain. Otoscopic examinations commonly reveal congestion of pars flaccida. Differences in Eustachian tube anatomy between adults and children result in more difficulty for reflux fluid invading the Eustachian tube and middle ear in adults, reducing the proportion of otitis media with effusion. However, diminished surfactant still alters the frequency and efficiency of Eustachian tube opening and closure, resulting in aural fullness or amplification of weak tinnitus signals. Laryngopharyngeal reflux can also cause tinnitus through the gut-brain axis. Recent researches have indicated that people with irritable bowel syndrome have amplified aberrant visceral perception. Investigations concerning visceral pain have indicated that nuclei involved in sensation include the anterior cingulate cortex, prefrontal cortex, and insular cortex. Laryngopharyngeal reflux is merely a symptom, and the particular pathophysiology is yet uncertain. Although loosened esophageal sphincter is undoubtedly the direct cause of reflux, muscular movement is also regulated by the neuroendocrine system and controlled by CNS. The complicated bidirectional interaction between the brain and the gut makes it difficult to identify whether CNS impacts intestinal function and produces reflux or intestinal dysfunction affects CNS, or they mutually influence each other. The gate control system of tinnitus principally involves the ventromedial prefrontal cortex (vmPFC) and the nucleus accumbens (NAcc) and includes the limbic system. Current researches have demonstrated a correlation between the gut microbiota and the limbic system; therefore the gate control system may be impacted by the gut microbiota. Improving the function of either the CNS or the gastrointestinal tract can reduce tinnitus.

11.7.3 Psychological Factors

11.7.3.1 Negative Emotions

The initial emotional response to hearing loss is a natural vigilance to anomalous noises, which can boost sympathetic nervous system excitability and strengthen the sensitivity of hair cells and the auditory central nervous system, thus improving auditory compensation effectiveness. However, consistently attributing negative connotations to tinnitus can lead to anxiety, tension, depression, and sleep disorders. This may overactivate the emotional system, rendering tinnitus a terrible experience. Controlling these unpleasant and inappropriate psychological responses is vital in the therapy of tinnitus.

11.7.3.2 Mental Disorders

The prevalence of mental diseases is particularly high among tinnitus patients, with the majority being affected by mood disorders, mainly depression and anxiety disorders. Most studies have indicated that 50–90% of tinnitus patients suffer from anxiety or depression, and there is a definite association between anxiety, depression, emotional qualities, and the intensity of tinnitus [11]. However, the degree of hearing loss seems unrelated to the severity of tinnitus. Although tinnitus is commonly accompanied by mental problems (particularly depression and anxiety), the exact causal link is not explicitly determined. Severe tinnitus can induce psychological discomfort, while the presence of depression and anxiety might diminish the patient's tolerance to tinnitus, thereby aggravating symptoms. In patients with tinnitus, a vicious cycle of tinnitus and mental stress is commonly observed; however, tinnitus is not necessarily the beginning element in this loop. Numerous researches have endeavored to study the correlation between mood disorders and tinnitus at the molecular level, claiming that the limbic system responsible for emotional and behavioral functions may be the underlying pathological substrate for both. Evidence reveals that the limbic systems of both individuals with tinnitus and those with anxiety are widely active and is potentially linked to the auditory system, which is the major cause of persistent severe tinnitus. Among tinnitus patients receiving placebo treatment, approximately 40% experience improved quality of life related to tinnitus, supporting the crucial regulatory function of psychological factors in the creation and exacerbation of tinnitus [12–16]. When tinnitus and mental illnesses overlap, both conditions should be treated simultaneously.

References

1. Chari DA, Limb CJ. Tinnitus. Med Clin North Am. 2018;102(6):1081–93.
2. Langguth B, Kreuzer PM, Kleinjung T, De Ridder D. Tinnitus: causes and clinical management. Lancet Neurol. 2013;12(9):920–30.
3. Friberg E, Jansson C, Mittendorfer-Rutz E, Rosenhall U, Alexanderson K. Sickness absence due to otoaudiological diagnoses and risk of disability pension: a nationwide Swedish prospective cohort study. PLoS One. 2012;7(1):e29966.
4. Pegge SAH, Steens SCA, Meijer FJA. Pulsatile tinnitus: differential diagnosis and radiological work-up. Insights Imaging. 2017;8(1):53–61.
5. Tunkel DE, Bauer CA, Sun GH, et al. Clinical practice guideline: tinnitus. Otolaryngol Head Neck Surg. 2014;151(2 Suppl):S1–S40.
6. Sindhusake D, Mitchell P, Newall P, et al. Prevalence and characteristics of tinnitus in older adults: the Blue Mountains Hearing Study. Int J Audiol. 2003;42(5):289–94.
7. McCormack A, Edmondson-Jones M, Somerset S, Hall D. A systematic review of the reporting of tinnitus prevalence and severity. Hear Res. 2016;337:70–9.
8. Nondahl DM, Cruickshanks KJ, Wiley TL, et al. Prevalence and 5-year incidence of tinnitus among older adults: the epidemiology of hearing loss study. J Am Acad Audiol. 2002;13(6):323–31.
9. Gopinath B, McMahon CM, Rochtchina E, Karpa MJ, Mitchell P. Incidence of tinnitus in older adults: the Blue Mountains Hearing Study. Ear Hear. 2010;31(3):407–12.
10. Nondahl DM, Cruickshanks KJ, Huang GH, et al. Tinnitus and its risk factors in the Beaver Dam Offspring Study. Int J Audiol. 2011;50(5):313–20.
11. Brueggemann P, Seydel C, Schaefer C, et al. ICD-10 symptom rating questionnaire for assessment of psychological comorbidities in patients with chronic tinnitus. HNO. 2019;67(Suppl 2):46–50.
12. Landgrebe M, Azevedo A, Baguley D, et al. Methodological aspects of clinical trials in tinnitus: a proposal for an international standard. J Psychosom Res. 2012;73(2):112–21.
13. Hesser H, Raggaset H, Andersson G. The effect of waiting: a meta-analysis of wait-list control groups in trials for tinnitus distress. J Psychosom Res. 2011;70(4):378–84.
14. Young C. What happens when people wait for therapy? Assessing the clinical significance of the changes observed over the waiting period for clients referred to a primary care psychology service. Prim Care Ment Health. 2006;4(2):113–9.
15. Posternak MA, Miller I. Untreated short-term course of major depression: a meta-analysis of outcomes from studies using wait-list control groups. J Affect Disord. 2001;66(2-3):139–46.
16. Devilly GJ, McFarlane AC. When wait lists are not feasible, nothing is a thing that does not need to be done. J Consult Clin Psychol. 2009;77(6):1159–68.

12 Classification Treatment of Subjective Tinnitus

Xin Ma, Qingyang Shi, and Lisheng Yu

12.1 The Current State of Treatment for Subjective Tinnitus

(1) Peculiar historical treatments. All disease treatments originate from an understanding of the underlying disease mechanisms. In the early, chaotic era of tinnitus comprehension, a myriad of unconventional therapies were employed, ranging from craniotomy, opium, cannabis, belladonna, purgatives, and various herbal remedies to bloodletting.

(2) Ear-directed therapies. For an extended period, it was widely believed that tinnitus stemmed from ear disorders. In 1924, sound masking therapy was proposed for tinnitus management. This treatment has evolved through numerous iterations of sound properties and continues to be used in clinical practice today [1]. However, the efficacy of masking is unpredictable due to its reliance on interactions between cochlear basilar membrane traveling waves, whereas tinnitus is not solely caused by vibrations of the basilar membrane. Cochlear nerve sectioning was also once attempted but showed only a 40% effectiveness rate, comparable to placebo, leading to its gradual abandonment.

(3) Combined treatment for both the ear and central nervous system. The most revolutionary advancement in understanding tinnitus came in the 1990s with the recognition of the central nervous system's role in its generation. It was realized that cochlear lesions serve as initiators of tinnitus, while the central nervous system's plastic responses to these lesions are the root cause. Emotional system involvement contributes to the chronicity of tinnitus. This insight has led to a plethora of treatments targeting chronic tinnitus, which currently form the mainstream international approach, encompassing four main aspects of comprehensive tinnitus management [2, 3]:

① Modifying sensory input: Primarily focusing on correcting or compensating for hearing loss accompanying tinnitus, this includes auditory training, sound therapy, hearing aids, music therapy, middle ear implants, cochlear implants, ear-specific treatments and surgeries, medications, and therapies aimed at improving inner ear function.

② Adjusting somatic sensory input for tinnitus management: Techniques such as trigger point therapy and acupuncture, as well as auricular cutaneous electrical stimulation.

X. Ma · Q. Shi · L. Yu (✉)
Department of Otorhinolaryngology, Head and Neck Surgery, People's Hospital, Peking University, Beijing, China
e-mail: 13581709195@164.com; 1710301204@pku.edu.cn

L. Yu (ed.), *Progress in Postauricular Administration*, Experts' Perspectives on Medical Advances, https://doi.org/10.1007/978-981-95-5102-6_12

③ Addressing maladaptive psychological reactions to tinnitus: It is not the condition itself but the individual's attitude and coping behavior that contribute to distress. Psychological interventions for adverse reactions to tinnitus primarily involve explanation and counseling, empowering patients with knowledge, advice, or support to foster positive psychological changes. These include relaxation techniques, mindfulness, hypnosis, and the widely recognized cognitive-behavioral therapy (CBT).

④ Central nervous system modulation therapies: Targeting excessive neural activity and frequency reorganization within the auditory cortex following peripheral auditory damage, which are implicated in tinnitus pathogenesis. Such treatments include repetitive transcranial magnetic stimulation (rTMS), electrical stimulation, and vagus nerve stimulation.

A concise overview of some representative treatment modalities is provided below:

12.1.1 Cognitive-Behavioral Therapy (CBT)

CBT has garnered favorable evaluations for tinnitus management. Originating from the field of psychotherapy, CBT aims to identify maladaptive cognitions and rectify negative thoughts through effective behavioral strategies. The CBT approach encompasses various components such as psychoeducation, counseling, relaxation training, behavioral reactivation, and mindfulness exercises. Widely applied in improving anxiety disorders, depression, insomnia, and managing health conditions related to unhealthy lifestyles like diabetes, obesity, and alcohol dependence, CBT is considered a gold standard in psychological treatments to a certain extent.

Since the 1980s, CBT has been utilized for tinnitus treatment, with American clinical practice guidelines recommending its referral to patients experiencing persistent and distressing tinnitus. The efficacy of CBT for tinnitus, particularly in cases of hyperacusis, stems from its ability to correct erroneous perceptions that lead to heightened sensitivity to tinnitus signals. Tinnitus loudness often surpasses hearing thresholds by only 5–10 dB, yet patients subjectively perceive it as louder, indicating a psychological acoustics phenomenon. Current perspectives suggest that CBT outperforms medication therapy and sound-based tinnitus therapies. Traditional tinnitus habituation therapy mainly relies on sound therapy, complemented by medical advice and psychological interventions. The goal of CBT is to diminish tinnitus sensitivity through specialized learning processes, potentially involving regular external stimuli, such as sound therapy. There is substantial evidence supporting the effectiveness of CBT in treating chronic and decompensated tinnitus, with two high-quality prospective controlled trials (graded as Level IIb evidence according to the Oxford classification) demonstrating significant differences in efficacy when comparing structured CBT to control groups using sound therapy alone. German recommendations advocate for combined medical-psychological interventions, emphasizing the role of cognitive-behavioral aspects. Moreover, CBT can be delivered remotely via the Internet, enhancing accessibility and implementation while maintaining comparable overall effectiveness to face-to-face CBT. However, research into CBT includes a multifaceted array of techniques, such as psychoeducation, cognitive reconstruction of dysfunctional beliefs, exposure techniques, mindfulness-based practices, stress reduction, and attention diversion tactics through exercise therapy, without true placebo controls or comparative "sham treatments." CBT incorporates relaxation therapy, which significantly impacts auditory perceptual disturbances characterized by tinnitus; however, this factor is noncontrollable and cannot be analyzed in isolation in outcome analyses. Studies often indicate that combining CBT with other treatments yields the best results. Although CBT has shown promise in improving quality of life, it does not alter tinnitus loudness or concurrent depression and must address coexisting fears, depression, sleep disturbances, and physiological factors influencing tinnitus intensity. Given that chronic, decompensated tinnitus represents a complex disorder, it requires intervention from otolaryngologists or psychologists trained in mental health and possibly an interdisciplinary team including audiologists and physiotherapists for comprehensive treatment. Treatment regimens should be grounded in evidence-based medicine (i.e., not chosen based on individual practitioners' preferences), implemented by specially trained therapists using standardized protocols, and evaluated using standardized methods.

12.1.2 Hearing Aid Therapy

Almost universally recommended by guidelines across nations, hearing aids are advocated for the treatment of tinnitus patients with accompanying hearing loss. Amplifying background sounds improves hearing and concurrently increases environmental noise, thereby narrowing the signal strength difference between tinnitus and ambient noise, reducing tinnitus loudness, and serving a therapeutic role in managing tinnitus. Furthermore, they can decrease the effort required to listen, enhance communication, and subsequently alleviate stress and anxiety. Some scholars hypothesize that hearing aids may exert physiological effects on brain activity related to tinnitus or prevent detrimental neuroplasticity triggered by auditory peripheral damage, potentially inducing "secondary" remodeling of the auditory system. However, due to the lack of high-level evidence, there is no consensus on whether hearing aids should be prescribed for individuals with mild hearing loss accompanied by tinnitus.

12.1.3 Masking Therapy

Masking tests demonstrate that if an individual's threshold at 1000 Hz is 0 dB, it shifts to 50 dB or 52 dB when exposed to a 50 dB white noise, simulating cochlear hearing loss, which underlies the mechanism of the Langenbeck audiometry test. This phenomenon is known as masking. The ability of tinnitus to be masked by sound stimulation represents a significant pathophysiological characteristic, and it also serves as a therapeutic approach, facilitating tinnitus classification. Ideal masking utilizes pure tones or narrowband noise, selected based on frequency matching results from tinnitus assessments. By incrementally increasing the intensity of a pure tone (or narrowband noise), the minimum intensity (minimum masking level, MML) that completely suppresses tinnitus can be determined. A graphical representation of the MMLs recorded in the form of an audiogram is referred to as a tinnitus masking audiogram, with Feldman categorizing them into convergent, divergent, overlapping, refractory, scattering, and diffuse types. Peripheral tinnitus responds well to masking therapy. However, for treating central tinnitus, a pure tone matching the tinnitus frequency must be used, with the volume exceeding the tinnitus by 20 dB, which patients often find intolerable. Excessive loudness could potentially cause noise-induced damage; thus, broadband noise therapy is now more commonly employed, the principles of which align with those of habituation therapy.

12.1.4 Tinnitus Retraining Therapy (TRT)

Proposed by Jastreboff and Hazell in 1993, the rationale of TRT is based on the premise that the primary origin of some tinnitus lies within the central auditory system, with chronic tinnitus often demonstrating a trend toward centralization. Thus, the therapeutic approach aims to decrease or eliminate the sensitivity of the central nervous system to tinnitus, essentially endeavoring to restore the filtering function of the auditory system and interrupt the auditory perception of tinnitus. TRT comprises partial tinnitus masking, relaxation techniques, distraction, and counseling from healthcare professionals. In foreign clinical settings, noise generators resembling behind-the-ear hearing aids are used to deliver sounds across various frequencies, or customized CDs, radios, tapes, etc. can be employed for training purposes to foster habituation to tinnitus. TRT necessitates a certain intensity and an extended treatment duration, typically involving 4–6 h per day over 1–2 years. It is crucial to maintain a volume just sufficient to reach the hearing threshold without being overly loud. While Jastreboff did not emphasize psychological counseling as a key aspect of TRT, recent evidence suggests that the core components of TRT—the noise generator or tinnitus sound therapy (inclusive of hearing aid plus tinnitus sound therapy)—do not significantly influence treatment outcomes, with the physician's advice being the most important part of TRT. Therefore, in the context of chronic tinnitus management, active cognitive interventions prove superior to passive treatments using tinnitus maskers.

12.1.5 Sound Therapy

Currently, several types of sound are utilized in clinical practice, including external noise or frequency-modulated sounds for tinnitus treatment, music therapy, and noise therapy. A meta-analysis encompassing 6 studies with a total of 553 patients concluded that there was no detectable improvement in tinnitus after treatment solely with external noise or amplified sounds (via hearing aids). Due to the multifaceted nature of these therapies, conclusive evidence-based medicine cannot be definitively drawn. However, compared to numerous pharmacological treatments, the advantage of sound therapy lies in its lack of side effects. The authors emphasize that the absence of clear evidence does not imply a lack of clinical efficacy; sound therapy should remain a component of a comprehensive treatment regimen for chronic tinnitus. The Nottingham research group led by Hoare and Hall has reviewed various combined therapies augmented with noise therapy for tinnitus. Fundamentally, the underlying concept of noise therapy posits that tinnitus alters cortical tension, leading to increased spontaneous activity in auditory pathway neurons, accompanied by emotional changes (network connections). Sound therapy is considered acoustic neuromodulation, employing individually tailored sound stimuli such as serenade (serenade therapy), frequency-modulated music (neuromonics), hearing aids with specialized soothing sounds (Widex Zen), or personalized sounds for auditory system training. Relatively few reliable studies exist regarding these sound-based treatment modalities, with only weak evidence supporting individualized frequency-based auditory training. Due to the dearth of efficacy evidence, more persuasive research has yet to be published.

Sweetow from San Francisco has pointed out that numerous studies on sound therapy are problematic and lack robust evidence. He introduced a novel music therapy approach employing intermittent tones, distinct from existing music that influences emotions. Implemented via hearing aids, this method not only addresses hearing loss but also possesses relaxing and ameliorative effects. Noise therapy constitutes a significant component of many habituation therapies, such as tinnitus retraining therapy (TRT), often accompanied by psychological support interventions. However, standalone sound therapy is generally considered insufficient, especially given its high cost which, when not covered by insurance providers, imposes an additional financial burden on tinnitus sufferers. Hoare et al.'s review reflects the current objective state of affairs yet underscores the need for more consistent and stable research evidence pertaining to both simple sound treatments and other sound-based methodologies, including so-called precision sound therapy targeted at the tinnitus frequency under the umbrella of "neuromodulation." To date, cohort studies have failed to conclusively demonstrate the efficacy of sound therapy when used in isolation. Sound therapy is commonly employed as part of a multifaceted or comprehensive treatment regimen rather than as a singular therapeutic modality.

12.1.6 Repetitive Transcranial Magnetic Stimulation (rTMS) Therapy

Repetitive transcranial magnetic stimulation is a diagnostic tool for cortical central nervous system disorders and can also serve therapeutic purposes. rTMS noninvasively examines and modulates local cortical excitability (as summarized by Hallett (2000)) [4]. A brief (100–300 ms) electromagnetic field (with an intensity of 1.5–2 Tesla) is generated through a coil placed on the scalp to activate cortical neurons. High-frequency stimulation (>10 Hz) can temporarily disrupt cortical function to assess its functionality, while low-frequency stimulation (<1 Hz) can reduce cortical activity in the targeted area, with application durations not exceeding 30 min. This serves as the theoretical foundation for using rTMS in treating chronic subjective tinnitus. However, there remains a dearth of substantial clinical research evidence regarding the feasibility, reliability, and effectiveness of this method.

12.1.7 Electrical Stimulation Therapy

Electrical stimulation techniques have been attempted to treat tinnitus for over two centuries, involving various methods such as transcutaneous, mastoid, tympanic cavity, promontory, and cochlear implants. Despite reports of variable efficacy, no prospective, controlled studies exist. Currently, neurosurgical approaches consider stimulating specific cortical regions to manage tinnitus, based on the premise that implanted cortical electrodes effectively alleviate phantom limb pain. Given the transient effects of rTMS on cortical excitability, precise, long-term electrical stimulation may potentially provide sustained tinnitus relief. rTMS is considered a noninvasive screening method prior to invasive electrical stimulation surgery. The specificity, reliability, efficacy, and feasibility of this tinnitus treatment are still debated, particularly concerning the impact of cortical electrical stimulation on excessive excitation and plasticity. For patients with severe hearing loss, cochlear implants can deliver effective electrical stimulation; however, it has yet to become a standard treatment option due to its narrow indication range, primarily for profound deafness cases.

12.1.8 Vagus Nerve Stimulation

Transcutaneous vagus nerve stimulation is considered a novel and promising approach for tinnitus management. Although initial findings were reported in animal experiments published in *Nature*, they carry significant medical implications. Animal studies show that when combined with training, electrically stimulating the vagus nerve allows for rapid learning. In treating human chronic tinnitus, it is hypothesized that concurrent sound therapy and direct vagus nerve stimulation could correct tinnitus symptoms. A prospective study involved 24 tinnitus patients who underwent 3–10 weeks of vagus nerve stimulation, accompanied by cardiac monitoring to assess safety and feasibility. Two cases of cardiac complications arose, suggesting that the treatment may lead to QRS complex shortening on ECG, although no arrhythmias were observed in otherwise healthy individuals. Another feasibility study from New Zealand investigated the application of this treatment in humans by implanting electrodes in the neck to stimulate the vagus nerve in ten tinnitus patients. Over a 20-day period, patients listened to sounds different from their tinnitus for 2.5 h daily while receiving vagus nerve stimulation. The treatment was well-tolerated without adverse effects, and the authors deemed it safe and feasible. One patient with severe, treatment-resistant tinnitus received an implanted vagus nerve stimulator in the cerebral cortex, followed by 4 weeks of sound therapy. There was improvement in THI scores and depression for 2 months, but symptoms returned to pretreatment levels thereafter. The authors argue that vagus nerve stimulation should be considered an efficacious treatment option.

12.1.9 Myofascial Trigger Point Treatment for Tinnitus

Myofascial trigger points (MTPs), typically associated with myofascial pain syndrome, have been explored in relation to tinnitus in a Brazilian study. MTPs often reside in postural muscles of the neck and shoulders. Among 94 tinnitus patients examined, 68 had at least 1 MTP identified, and half experienced tinnitus reduction following MTP stimulation. This result aligns with previous discussions on the interplay between craniofacial trigeminal nerves and auditory nerves and the concept of somatosensory tinnitus, which is often recognized as a distinct subtype in various tinnitus classifications. Identifying and targeting these sensitive trigger points holds significance if patients report their presence and influence on their tinnitus.

12.1.10 Pharmacological Treatment for Chronic Tinnitus

Despite numerous trials on tinnitus medications, no guidelines currently recommend a specific drug for chronic tinnitus treatment. While some drugs demonstrate effectiveness for certain tinnitus patients, their benefits cannot be consistently replicated across other patients, indicating that medications are not ineffective but rather necessitate a more nuanced categorization of tinnitus, with different subtypes responding favorably to specific drugs.

12.1.11 Surgical Treatment

For select cases of objective tinnitus, especially venous pulsatile tinnitus originating from the middle ear or mastoid, surgical intervention can be considered. However, surgery is not the primary choice for treating subjective tinnitus. Historically, destructive surgeries targeting the inner ear or auditory nerve have largely been abandoned despite offering short-term benefits due to high recurrence rates. Presently, surgeries mainly focus on addressing tinnitus caused by vascular loops compressing the auditory nerve. The procedure involves decompression of the vascular loop, a technique used for hemifacial spasm and trigeminal neuralgia. Decompression surgeries targeting the eighth cranial nerve for tinnitus yield poor long-term outcomes and are not routinely recommended. Following surgery for chronic suppurative otitis media, approximately one-third of patients experience tinnitus relief, one-third remain unchanged, and another third report increased tinnitus severity, indicating that middle ear surgery does not significantly resolve tinnitus issues. For Meniere's disease, endolymphatic sac decompression results in tinnitus improvement in about half of the patients.

The current state of tinnitus treatment presents two main challenges: first, a lack of refined classification systems for tinnitus, and second, the tendency to view tinnitus as solely a symptom—a warning signal of underlying health issues—while insufficient attention is given to the role of nonauditory system diseases in its development. To address these challenges, tinnitus needs to be classified multidimensionally based on duration, severity, and physiological factors, as detailed in the subsequent chapter. The plethora of available treatments highlights the heterogeneous nature of tinnitus, where therapies effective for one patient may not generalize to others. Attempting all treatments for every patient can lead to multiple failures and dissatisfaction, emphasizing the need for a more tailored, evidence-based approach to tinnitus management.

12.2 Classification of Subjective Tinnitus

Tinnitus is bifurcated into two principal categories: objective and subjective tinnitus, with distinct treatment approaches. This text primarily focuses on the latter, as it is significantly more prevalent than its objective counterpart, albeit with less clarity regarding its etiology and pathophysiology, leading to suboptimal therapeutic outcomes.

Subjective tinnitus is a pervasive global issue, as McCormack A's review (1980–2015) indicates an incidence ranging from 5.1% to 42.7%, escalating with age and noise exposure. About 25% of individuals with tinnitus report that it impacts their daily life, with 1–3% experiencing severe impairment. The rate of work absence due to tinnitus triples that of other health conditions, and suicide risk among tinnitus patients is tenfold higher compared to nontinnitus populations.

Despite its high prevalence, tinnitus remains a challenging therapeutic conundrum worldwide, characterized by substantial interindividual variability. Firstly, different patients exhibit distinct tinnitus characteristics, such as pulsatile versus nonpulsatile, intermittent versus continuous, unilateral versus bilateral, varying pitch and intensity, responsiveness to external noise, and alterations in tone and nature with head and neck muscle movements. Secondly, there is considerable variation in whether tinnitus can be masked among different patients. Thirdly, accompanying comorbidities differ greatly across individuals with tinnitus, including the degree and type of hearing loss, presence or absence of hyperacusis, vertigo, headaches, anxiety, depression, and other affective disorders. Fourthly, and most crucially, individual responses to identical tinnitus treatment regimens vary significantly. Biesinger et al. (1998) documented nearly 60 distinct treatments used for chronic idiopathic tinnitus, and since then, the number of treatment methods has continued to grow [5]. While many patients derive benefits, a treatment efficacious for one patient may prove entirely ineffective for another. For instance, sound therapy for tinnitus alleviates symptoms for some yet exacerbates them in others when exposed to noisy environments. Similarly, carbamazepine, an anticonvulsant, has shown mixed results; while some trials yield negative outcomes, it demonstrates positive effects on "typist" type tinnitus. These observations underscore that the underlying mechanisms driving tinnitus are highly divergent among different patients. Without proper classification, applying uniform treatments to all tinnitus patients is unlikely to yield satisfactory outcomes, contributing significantly to the lack of success in pharmacological trials targeting tinnitus. Selecting patients with specific tinnitus attributes for tailored therapies could potentially enhance treatment efficacy. The classification of tinnitus patients has long been a topic of significant interest. Past literature has proposed multiple categorization schemes based on factors such as disease duration, severity of tinnitus, tinnitus features, masking properties, auditory status, psychological state, somatosensory components, and presence of hyperacusis, among others. This chapter provides an overview of those classification methods with substantial clinical relevance, aiming to offer guidance for tinnitus diagnosis and management.

12.2.1 Categorization of Tinnitus by Duration

Categorizing tinnitus based on its duration is a crucial aspect in the management of this condition. Acute and chronic tinnitus exhibit distinct therapeutic strategies, as evidenced by numerous studies that draw parallels between tinnitus and pain, with the latter being more extensively researched. Acute and chronic pain differ significantly in etiology, pathogenesis, pathophysiology, symptomatology, diagnosis, and treatment. Acute pain serves as an alarm signal indicative of bodily harm, whereas chronic pain itself constitutes a disease entity, often characterized by false alarms not reflecting actual tissue damage. Analogously, acute tinnitus functions as a symptom—a warning bell necessitating active investigation into its cause, while chronic tinnitus represents a standalone disease. Hence, classifying tinnitus according to its duration is vital for devising appropriate treatment strategies and predicting outcomes.

Different national guidelines have demarcated primary tinnitus into acute and chronic phases using timeframes of 3 months (as per Japanese guidelines) and 6 months as the threshold between the two stages. However, this temporal cutoff presents a clinical drawback, imposing a sense of urgency on both patients and physicians. The perception that tinnitus persisting beyond 6 months is unlikely to resolve can generate considerable psychological stress, which, in turn, may exacerbate tinnitus symptoms through increased attention and anxiety. Longitudinal research indicates that among 481 individuals presenting with tinnitus at baseline assessment, 81.6% (346 cases) still experienced tinnitus after 5 years, suggesting a natural remission rate of approximately 20%. Although the study did not categorize tinnitus history, it predominantly comprised chronic cases. Notably, severity levels fluctuated over time; initially mild tinnitus progressed to moderate in 39.6% and severely affected in 5.9%, while over half of those initially experiencing severe tinnitus reported improvement, with 51.8% becoming moderate and 3.6% mild. Overall, about half of tinnitus sufferers experienced some degree of improvement with prolonged duration.

The delineation between acute and chronic tinnitus could be more rationalized by considering insights from tinnitus pathogenesis. It is currently hypothesized that tinnitus arises due to decreased peripheral auditory system activity following cochlear damage, leading to a downregulation of inhibitory function within the central cortex. This results in hyperexcitability and neural synchronization across the central auditory system, including various auditory cortices, accompanied by disarray in tonotopic organization and heightened neuronal activity around the impaired frequency range. A widely accepted view posits that although cochlear abnormalities may initiate tinnitus, the subsequent series of changes within the central nervous system are responsible for its persistence. This process is termed auditory central reorganization, suggesting that tinnitus can be conceptualized as a "central plasticity disorder." In instances such as noise-induced hearing loss or sudden sensorineural hearing loss, tinnitus typically emerges concurrently. Within such a short timeframe, the central changes primarily involve alterations in synaptic efficiency. Over time, structural changes gradually develop in the central nervous system, and once established, reversing these changes becomes challenging regardless of the initial trigger. Research utilizing repetitive transcranial magnetic stimulation (rTMS) reveals that networks involved in tinnitus are different for patients with tinnitus lasting over 4 years compared to those with less than 4 years, with even functional connectivity showing marked differences within similar regions. While the progression from morphological to structural changes in the central nervous system occurs gradually with individual variability, a practical cutoff point of 4 years might be useful for clinicians to distinguish between acute and chronic tinnitus. During the initial 4-year period, addressing the underlying causes and correcting centrally generated functional alterations may provide a window of opportunity for reversal. Furthermore, this extended timeline alleviates the sense of urgency, potentially preventing heightened anxiety associated with tinnitus and the vicious cycle it engenders. Although current evidence supporting a 4-year threshold is limited, longitudinal follow-ups suggest that most tinnitus cases following sudden deafness show significant improvement within 1 year, thus rendering at least 1 year as a more reasonable boundary for distinguishing between acute and chronic tinnitus than the traditional 6-month mark.

12.2.2 Tinnitus Severity Grading Through Questionnaires

Tinnitus, being a purely subjective sensation, necessitates the use of self-report questionnaires as vital assessment tools. To date, more than 20 such questionnaires have been employed globally in clinical settings, including the Tinnitus Questionnaire (TQ), Tinnitus Handicap Inventory (THI), Tinnitus Reaction Questionnaire (TRQ), Tinnitus Handicap Questionnaire (THQ), and Tinnitus Functional Index (TFI), among others. These questionnaires encompass multiple domains, such as emotional impact, attentional disruption, sleep disturbances, auditory perceptual difficulties, interference with daily activities or work, and patients' attitudes toward tinnitus, thereby effectively evaluating psychological characteristics of tinnitus sufferers. Researchers and clinicians have translated these tinnitus questionnaires—including but not limited to the aforementioned measures—into various languages, enabling them to grade the severity of tinnitus across patient populations. Specifically, five English-language tinnitus measurement questionnaires have been translated and validated into Mandarin Chinese versions, which include two iterations of THI1 and THI2, THQ, Tinnitus Activities Questionnaire (TAQ), and the Tinnitus

Questionnaire (TQ). Notably, the THI, developed by Newman et al. in 1996, is the most widely used self-assessment questionnaire for tinnitus worldwide, designed to assess the impact of tinnitus on patients' quality of life. This 25-item instrument is divided into three sections, Function (12 items), Emotion (8 items), and Catastrophic Reactions (5 items), each probing physical functioning, psychological distress, feelings of despair, and loss of control. The THI has been recognized as a useful screening tool for comorbid psychiatric conditions.

The 2012 Chinese Consensus on Tinnitus recommends the use of tinnitus evaluation questionnaires that categorize tinnitus into six distinct grades, differentiating between intermittent and continuous tinnitus while also considering the degree of impairment caused by the condition. Although the physiological aspects of tinnitus may vary minimally among chronic tinnitus patients, with matched loudness tests revealing tinnitus sounds typically above threshold by 5–10 dB, such tests do not provide a graded measure of tinnitus severity. This suggests that the physiological factors contributing to tinnitus are relatively consistent across individuals, whereas the differences primarily lie in psychological factors, which have been extensively detailed earlier in the discussion.

12.2.3 Classification of Tinnitus Based on Physiological Mechanisms

Referencing the previous section on physiological factors of tinnitus, it can be categorized into audiological-related tinnitus subtypes: (1) acute hearing loss-associated tinnitus, (2) fluctuating hearing loss-related tinnitus, and (3) chronic symmetric moderate-to-severe hearing loss-associated tinnitus. Additionally, there are regulatory system-related tinnitus types, including menopause-related tinnitus in women, anxiety or depression-linked tinnitus, tinnitus associated with obstructive sleep apnea-hypopnea syndrome, and reflux-related tinnitus, each presenting distinct characteristics that allow for the gradual identification of specific features and subsequent targeted treatment strategies. There also exist idiopathic cases of tinnitus where no clear contributing factors are identified, and these patients often respond poorly to empirical treatments. Therefore, further exploration of potential etiologies is necessary. As our understanding expands, the prevalence of such idiopathic cases is expected to decline.

Regarding tinnitus management, the duration of symptoms informs treatment strategy and prognosis, while severity grading dictates the necessity of psychological intervention. Mechanism-based classification plays a crucial role in identifying physiological factors and directing tailored treatments. It is noteworthy that while tinnitus is predominantly benign in most instances, certain cases warrant immediate attention to exclude potentially dangerous causes. Advanced imaging techniques have made diagnosing tumors or central nervous system disorders relatively straightforward; thus, diagnostic tests not only rule out severe illnesses but also provide reassurance to patients, particularly those with anxiety traits. Furthermore, tinnitus accompanied by suicidal ideation should be considered a high-risk variant and prompt referral to appropriate specialists is recommended.

12.3 Recommended Treatment Process for Subjective Tinnitus

In the medical context, tinnitus management is often stratified into three tiers: primary prevention, secondary etiological treatment, and tertiary symptomatic management. Historically, tinnitus has largely been treated symptomatically with suboptimal outcomes. The most optimal approach for clinicians is to diligently search for and identify underlying causes (precipitants) and implement targeted etiological interventions while educating patients about the cause(s) of their tinnitus to prevent recurrence or exacerbation. In this process, a thorough history-taking holds paramount importance.

12.3.1 History taking

The structured questioning in the patient's history should encompass both the characteristics of tinnitus and its severity.

12.3.1.1 Structured Inquiry into Tinnitus Characteristics

This aspect significantly aids in determining the etiology, precipitants, and prognosis of tinnitus, warranting meticulous inquiry. While acute tinnitus may be triggered by a single factor such as hearing loss, chronic cases often involve multiple causative factors or triggers. The questioning should systematically explore three domains:

(1) Auditory system: Pertaining to any issues that could contribute to peripheral auditory dysfunction
(2) Central nervous system: Investigating potential central nervous system involvement or modulation contributing to tinnitus perception.
(3) Eustachian tube function: Assessing the role of eustachian tube dysfunction in relation to tinnitus development

This comprehensive approach to tinnitus assessment aims to provide a more informed basis for subsequent therapeutic decisions tailored to individual patients' unique presentations and etiologies.

Tinnitus precipitants encompass hearing loss, sleep disturbances, stress, emotional factors, trauma, and Eustachian tube dysfunction, among others. The inquiry into sleep patterns is of utmost importance due to the bidirectional relationship between tinnitus and sleep disorders, with the latter being a leading cause of chronic tinnitus.

Characteristics of tinnitus include tonality, frequency, and persistence (continuous vs. intermittent). Tinnitus resulting from external or middle ear pathologies often manifests as low-to-middle-frequency sounds. In the cochlea, there exists a precise tonotopic organization where the basal turn processes high frequencies while the apical turn is responsible for lower frequencies. Hence, depending on the site of inner ear damage, tinnitus can be perceived as either low or high frequency. The auditory nerve also has a defined tonotopic organization, with the periphery responsive to high frequencies and the mid-section to low frequencies; thus, auditory nerve pathology typically presents as high-frequency tinnitus. When a vascular loop exerts pressure near the auditory nerve, a characteristic high-frequency pulsatile "buzzing" sound may ensue.

The onset time of tinnitus is currently demarcated at 6 months as the threshold between acute and chronic phases, albeit with some controversy. A detailed discussion regarding this classification in relation to tinnitus treatment strategies is presented in the chapter dedicated to tinnitus categorization and management.

Tinnitus laterality and frequency: Unilateral/bilateral or cerebral tinnitus? Are bilateral tinnitus symptoms synchronous in frequency? In cases where bilateral tinnitus is synchronous, central involvement is more likely, given the strict tonotopic organization in the periphery; it is challenging to envision simultaneous peripheral damage at identical locations on both sides. Cerebral tinnitus is of central origin. The auditory cortex also exhibits tonotopic organization, with distinct low-frequency and high-frequency regions. Consequently, cerebral tinnitus can present as low- or high-pitched sounds. Rustling or hissing cerebral tinnitus often corresponds to cortical blood flow sounds, indicative of heightened cortical excitability. Bilateral tinnitus can be either synchronous or asynchronous in frequency. Bilateral synchronous tinnitus, as well as cerebral tinnitus, frequently suggests underlying brainstem or cortical pathologies or functional abnormalities. Due to the function of the acoustic crossover, severe symptoms in one side may actually indicate pathology in the contralateral central region. Bilateral asynchronous tinnitus or unilateral tinnitus presenting with multiple sound types points to the presence of diverse pathophysiological mechanisms. Tinnitus typically manifests as meaningless sounds; however, when it presents as meaningful speech or musical hallucinations, it is often associated with psychiatric disorders.

Onset pattern: sudden versus gradual onset?

Temporal patterns and triggers of tinnitus modulation: The conditions under which tinnitus exacerbates or alleviates are crucial to document. Changes in tinnitus intensity during head and neck movements, as well as temporomandibular joint activities, may provide diagnostic clues. If tinnitus worsens during chewing or eating, an external auditory canal foreign body such as hair or impacted earwax on the tympanic membrane should be initially considered. Diet-related tinnitus, due to its delayed onset, is often overlooked by patients. A worsening of tinnitus when speaking loudly or engaging in physical activity might suggest a link to gastroesophageal reflux. Some patients report increased tinnitus while combing their hair or clenching their jaws; the presence of trigger points on the scalp that modulate tinnitus upon pressure indicates neural connections between peripheral skin and auditory pathways. Notably, the central auditory cortex is unique among sensory cortices for maintaining connections with peripheral sensations. In certain cases, profoundly deaf individuals experience numbness or loss of sensation around the ears.

Modulation of tinnitus in noisy versus quiet environments: An exacerbation of tinnitus in noisy settings, often accompanied by hyperacusis, frequently associates with migraine or central sensitization syndromes.

Relationship with emotions, sleep, and headaches: The cooccurrence of tinnitus with other symptoms, including hearing loss, dizziness, headaches, aural fullness, hyperacusis, and the subsequent emotional and sleep disturbances, must be carefully assessed. For instance, tinnitus accompanied by hyperacusis should prompt consideration of a diagnosis involving migraines or central sensitization syndrome.

Previous medical history: This includes a history of hearing loss, headaches, dizziness, sleep disturbances, psychiatric disorders, menopause, obstructive sleep apnea syndrome (OSAS), thyroid function abnormalities, rhinitis and sinusitis, laryngopharyngeal reflux disease, and previous treatment history for tinnitus.

12.3.1.2 Tinnitus Questionnaires

These tools serve to accurately determine the severity of tinnitus, with particular emphasis on identifying cases accompanied by severe psychological disorders that necessitate prompt referral to specialized care. Refer to the previous chapter on tinnitus classification for further details. The use of the Tinnitus Handicap Inventory (THI) and the six-level classification from the 2012 Tinnitus Consensus is recommended, whereupon patients with severe tinnitus should be promptly referred, and those at level 4 or above are considered for psychological interventions.

12.3.2 Clinical Otological Evaluation

- Otoscopy to exclude outer and middle ear pathologies. Otoscopic examination provides more comprehensive information than tympanometry.
- Nasal endoscopy to assess the Eustachian tube and nasopharyngeal region for conditions that might impair Eustachian tube function, including gastroesophageal reflux and laryngopharyngeal reflux disease.

Auscultation: This checks for signs of carotid artery stenosis; vertebral-basilar insufficiency can sometimes be detected through auscultation of the neck and posterior auricular areas. Tinnitus exacerbated by neck movement or compression may indicate a venous origin.

12.3.3 Ancillary Examinations and Current Clinical Applications

(1) Audiological assessments: Alongside standard tests such as pure-tone audiometry, tympanometry, otoacoustic emissions, and auditory brainstem response testing, specific examinations for tinnitus include tone and frequency matching, loudness assessment,

masking properties evaluation, residual inhibition testing, and uncomfortable loudness levels. However, the American Tinnitus Guidelines suggest that meticulous tinnitus-specific tests may not always be necessary for chronic cases.

(2) Imaging studies: Depending on the clinical presentation, imaging investigations may encompass cranial, internal auditory canal, sinus, and ear radiographic evaluations. In cases of asymmetric hearing loss, an MRI of the internal auditory canal is recommended. For acute tinnitus patients presenting with headaches, facial numbness, or other abnormal sensations, urgent cranial imaging, particularly MRI of the internal auditory canal and skull base, is advised. Although the vast majority of tinnitus patients do not have central nervous system lesions, such imaging can offer reassurance to patients who are concerned about intracranial tumors or vascular abnormalities, reducing anxiety and, in some instances, becoming part of the therapeutic process itself.

(3) Tinnitus-related factor investigations: When tinnitus is suspected to be associated with regulatory mechanisms, a systemic examination is required. Currently, this often involves selecting appropriate blood tests, sleep apnea monitoring, and hormonal assessments according to the patient's condition, which may include female sex hormone panels or testosterone levels in males, among others.

(4) Psychiatric disorders and sleep questionnaires: Assessment of mental health status is also of great importance, as previously introduced in the context of tinnitus classification. After an initial evaluation with the THI, patients with a severity level of 4 or above are recommended to undergo psychological and sleep state assessments. This serves two purposes: to provide a basis for clinical medication decisions and to educate patients about the multifaceted nature of their tinnitus, emphasizing both physiological and psychological components.

Other brain functional imaging modalities, such as positron emission tomography (PET) scans, are predominantly utilized in research settings and are often challenging to implement in routine practice.

Following the thorough history-taking and examination process, the following five objectives should be achieved:

(1) Differentiate between subjective and objective tinnitus, each requiring distinct diagnostic and treatment pathways.
(2) Diagnose certain conditions associated with tinnitus, such as impacted earwax, otitis media, Meniere's disease, and vestibular migraine (VM), among others.
(3) Exclude central nervous system disorders, auditory nerve tumors, and nasopharyngeal malignancies through imaging studies.
(4) Recognize tinnitus accompanied by suicidal ideation as a high-risk variant, necessitating prompt referral to appropriate specialists.
(5) Identify patients with acute tinnitus accompanying acute hearing loss, which, while not life-threatening, constitutes an urgent otological emergency requiring expedited management.

Upon completion of these preliminary evaluations, the majority of tinnitus cases prove to be benign. Emphasizing this point during positive counseling is crucial. Subsequent treatment involves categorizing tinnitus according to its acute or chronic nature. Acute tinnitus is viewed as a symptom—a warning signal indicating functional issues within the body; hence, the primary focus is on actively identifying and addressing physiological causes. Conversely, chronic tinnitus is considered a standalone disease entity, often characterized by "false alarms" despite no underlying pathology. Therefore, the main therapeutic goal in chronic tinnitus is to cease the false alerts and elevate the threshold for triggering tinnitus sensations.

12.3.4 Acute Tinnitus Management

Currently, numerous treatments for tinnitus primarily target chronic cases, yet all chronic tinnitus arises from acute episodes. The American Tinnitus Association guidelines suggest that due to the potential for spontaneous resolution in acute tinnitus, a period of observation can be warranted. However, it remains challenging to predict which acute cases will resolve spontaneously and which will progress to chronicity. As previously mentioned, those with acute tinnitus who do not seek medical attention are more likely to experience self-resolution, whereas patients presenting with acute tinnitus often exhibit heightened anxiety regarding their symptoms. Therefore, a proactive approach toward managing acute tinnitus is crucial; only through timely and appropriate management of acute cases can the progression to chronicity be effectively prevented.

12.3.4.1 When encountering patients with acute tinnitus

A diligent search for its etiology should be undertaken. Historically, the focus on identifying tinnitus causes has largely been confined to the auditory system, leading to a high proportion of idiopathic cases. Given the introduction of the tinnitus regulatory system and associated factors, the search for causative elements should now extend beyond acute auditory system pathologies to encompass various factors potentially affecting the tinnitus control system, as detailed in the chapter on physiological aspects of tinnitus.

12.3.4.2 For patients where no clear physiological cause for tinnitus can be identified

Treatment regimens analogous to those used for sudden sensorineural hearing loss (SSHL) may be employed. Regardless of whether the tinnitus is of high or low frequency, administration of high-dose corticosteroids, such as 1mg/kg body weight/day, is recommended. Treatment decisions should be individualized based on patient-specific factors, including treatment preference, level of distress, and the presence of accompanying symptoms like hearing loss. Acute tinnitus pharmacotherapy can follow SSHL treatment paradigms, considering the use of monotherapy or combination therapy with the following interventions: corticosteroids, rheological blood modifiers, and ion-based treatments (such as lidocaine).

12.3.4.3 Placebo treatment

The array of tinnitus treatment modalities seems to yield some degree of efficacy, with placebo effects playing a significant role. From a psychological standpoint, numerous mechanisms contribute to the placebo response, including expectation, conditioning, learning, memory, motivation, somatic focus, reward, and anxiety reduction. Among these, two principal mechanisms—subject expectancy and classical conditioning—are likely paramount; however, placebo effects extend beyond psychological dimensions, involving changes in neurotransmitter activity within the brain. For instance, the placebo effect in pain management is often attributed to the release of endogenous opioids such as endorphins. Extensive evidence suggests that placebo responses across different diseases can be mediated by various mechanisms, leading to the release of distinct neurotransmitters and neuromodulators. In Parkinson's disease, placebo treatments can induce dopamine release and alterations in neuronal firing in the striatum, basal ganglia, and thalamus. The nucleus accumbens, which influences the perception of pleasure and reward, has been proposed by A Rolls as a potential source of the placebo effect. He posits that heightened activation in certain brain regions due to positive expectations represents the body's coping mechanism against illness, and when positive expectations activate the reward system, immune function may also be enhanced—a potential evolutionary advantage. Given the involvement of the nucleus accumbens in the tinnitus gating system and its relevance to drug addiction and placebo effects, administering a placebo therapy tailored to the patient's characteristics and cultural background could be considered a viable treatment option for acute tinnitus.

12.3.4.4 Emphasizing the role of the emotional system in acute tinnitus onset

The emotional system plays a pivotal role in the progression of tinnitus from acute to chronic stages. When faced with a nonlife-threatening symptom like tinnitus, many patients initially attempt to attribute their symptoms to factors such as diet, exercise routines, medication use, or preexisting health conditions. If they fail to find plausible explanations or experience unsatisfactory results, psychological reactions tend to intensify. Heightened psychological reactivity can lead patients to hyperfocus on their tinnitus, amplifying its perceived intensity and potentially triggering additional somatic symptoms, such as ear numbness, heaviness in the head, or even earache or headache, prompting medical consultation. Most patients place great hope in the initial encounter with their physician, expecting a reasonable explanation for their symptoms, clear and specific management strategies, and a favorable prognosis. The information and answers received from the doctor during the first visit significantly influence the patient's subsequent psychological development and the efficacy of treating their tinnitus symptomatology. Patients not only interpret the doctor's verbal expressions but also absorb the conveyed knowledge, confidence, and attitude through the physician's demeanor, conduct, and speech. During consultations, it is crucial to be cognizant of the patient's psychological profile, ensuring that all communication and behavior build trust and instill confidence in the improvement of tinnitus symptoms. In clinical practice, it is common to observe primary care physicians inadvertently conveying a lack of control or understanding of tinnitus, which can have detrimental psychological impacts on patients. Such careless language exacerbates anxiety about tinnitus rather than alleviating it and may erode the patient's confidence in the possibility of symptom improvement. Psychological interventions for acute tinnitus patients should primarily encompass the following aspects (further details would follow here based on the original text but are not provided).

(1) Providing an explanation of tinnitus generation: It is essential to inform patients that tinnitus does not arise spontaneously but has a physiological basis, akin to the pain experienced after a hand injury. Tinnitus serves as a gentle reminder of a bodily condition, which is often benign; thus, it necessitates undergoing certain investigations such as MRI scans to exclude potentially serious conditions. Once these have been ruled out, patients can be reassured that the issue is relatively minor.

(2) The resolution of tinnitus takes time: Disappearance of tinnitus typically occurs over a period measured in seasons (i.e., 3 months), and patience is required for its gradual diminishment. During this phase, patients should refrain from excessive attention to their tinnitus, as the brain assesses whether the tinnitus signal represents a danger or not. If the alarm persists without other concurrent issues, the brain may eventually reclassify tinnitus as a nonthreatening signal and diminish its presence. Overmonitoring the tinnitus could lead the brain to interpret the signal as threatening and thereby sustain it. Patients are advised against extensive online research, as information on tinnitus treatments tends to be skewed negatively due to the underrepresentation of self-resolving cases, leading to inherent biases.

(3) Avoidance strategies should not be excessive: Overly avoiding situations that trigger tinnitus inadvertently increases subconscious focus on it. Patients are encouraged to desist from deliberate avoidance behaviors like staying away from quiet environments, as these actions are counterproductive to tinnitus resolution. When experiencing intense tinnitus, mindfulness techniques or the introduction of background noise, including sound therapy, can be beneficial.

(4) Managing anxiety in high-risk patients: Individuals with anxiety tendencies are at higher risk for tinnitus chronicity. Alongside psychological support, these patients require appropriate anxiolytic medication. While traditional Chinese medicines may have a slower onset, SSRIs, SNRIs, and drugs like

Deanxit and benzodiazepines are commonly used. For patients with event-related anxiety stemming from tinnitus but without significant depressive symptoms and no contraindications, Deanxit or Lorazepam may be prescribed for a 2–4-week course, with the possibility of tapering off if tinnitus improves. In cases where anxiety symptoms are severe and discontinuation within a short timeframe is unlikely, the addition of Sertraline and Escitalopram to Deanxit may be considered, generally followed by discontinuing Deanxit after 2–3 weeks. SNRIs are also worth exploring, given their indication for neuropathic pain and the similarities between tinnitus and chronic pain. Ear specialists must thoroughly study drug inserts and potential side effects before prescribing these medications, starting with low doses. Moreover, when patients exhibit extreme anxiety, prompt referral to psychiatric specialists for collaborative treatment is recommended. An illustrative case involves a patient with acute tinnitus for 2 months, preceded by emotional stress, presenting with symmetric normal hearing bilaterally. It was hypothesized that the emotional event had affected the tinnitus regulatory system, resulting in acute tinnitus. After explaining the cause of tinnitus and considering the patient's anxiety, medications like Deanxit, Lorazepam, and Ginkgo extract were prescribed. At 1-month follow-up, the patient reported minimal improvement, although questionnaire scores showed slight progress. Another month of medication was prescribed, yet at the next visit, the patient expressed frustration and disappointment as there was still limited improvement despite adherence to the regimen. This experience highlighted the importance of addressing patient concerns, understanding the disease progression, fostering realistic expectations, and combining medication with psychoeducation for optimal outcomes in tinnitus management.

(5) Acute tinnitus patients often experience a degree of anxiety and tension, which is a natural protective response to sudden changes in their condition. However, a decline in anxiety levels over time is expected; persistence or rebound of anxiety beyond an appropriate timeframe initiates involvement of nonauditory systems, as previously discussed, and this process becomes independent of the initial auditory damage. Instead, it is governed by the central emotional system's ability to regulate and adapt to unexpected events. If patients continue to experience discomfort 3 months post-onset of acute tinnitus symptoms, it suggests a potential for tinnitus chronicity, resembling an adjustment disorder.

12.3.5 Subacute Tinnitus (Duration: 3 months to 1 year)

Germany has previously introduced the concept of subacute tinnitus. As mentioned earlier, the categorization of chronic tinnitus based on a relatively short duration is somewhat arbitrary. Subacute tinnitus cases can be managed using the four-tiered treatment approach for acute tinnitus; however, it is crucial to note that as the history lengthens, psychological interventions become increasingly important. Appropriate testing and positive interpretation are vital in this context.

12.3.6 Chronic Tinnitus (Duration > 1 year)

For chronic subjective tinnitus, it is essential to differentiate between compensatory and decompensated forms.

12.3.6.1 Compensatory tinnitus

This refers to tinnitus that is mild and tolerable, with patients not experiencing cognitive distractions, memory decline, sleep disturbances, headaches, hyperarousal, depression, or other neuropsychiatric symptoms. These individuals constitute about 90% of chronic tinnitus cases and can be considered "tinnitus bearers" rather than "patients." In the previous chapter's classification of acute and chronic tinnitus, structural changes in the central nervous system were discussed for cases exceeding 4 years. Reversing such changes becomes an arduous and lengthy process. However, for those with a shorter history (<4 years), addressing relevant physiological factors can still yield some therapeutic benefits. Our department collaborated with gynecology to investigate tinnitus in perimenopausal women, where 30% experienced tinnitus, primarily intermittent and mild. After receiving hormonal therapy, many reported disappearance of their tinnitus, indicating genuine loudness modification and resolution. Hence, for these tinnitus bearers with less extensive histories, targeting physiological factors is appropriate. However, for those with longer histories, realistic expectations should be set. Nonetheless, due to their relative lack of excessive concern over tinnitus, a positive explanation allows them to accept and coexist with tinnitus, much like they do with age spots or gray hair.

12.3.6.2 Decompensated tinnitus

This category includes severe tinnitus that patients find unbearable, accompanied by cognitive distractions, memory impairment, sleep disorders, anxiety, depression, and other neuropsychiatric symptoms. These are the true chronic tinnitus patients whose condition significantly impacts social functioning and necessitates serious intervention. In such instances, the tinnitus alarm function is significantly diminished, often involving "false alarms" resulting from central hypersensitivity to normal brain electrical signals. To manage these patients, the first step is to adjust the alarm mechanism to prevent oversensitivity. Secondarily, one must address physiological factors, as the initiating factors may no longer be crucial, while changes within the central nervous system play a more significant role in the progression of chronic tinnitus.

(1) Cognitive behavioral therapy (CBT): Correcting patients' misconceptions is pivotal to breaking the vicious cycle of central tinnitus. An active CBT approach, such as TDT (targeted diagnostic and treatment), is generally more effective than passive treatments like traditional TRT (tinnitus retraining therapy) that solely rely on sound masking. Providing accurate explanations about tinnitus mechanisms and offering a positive interpretation is particularly challenging in the management of chronic decompensated tinnitus. Convincing somatically focused tinnitus patients to accept that tinnitus results from central functional changes and involves excessive participation of psychological factors, and adhering to the treatment plan, is difficult. A systematic and professional cognitive-behavioral process is required, which our team is currently refining and aims to share insights into treating chronic decompensated tinnitus later.
(2) Central sensitization management: This concept has been around for some time and was introduced earlier. Drug treatment mainly comprises antiepileptic medications and antidepressants/anxiolytics, emphasizing adequate dosage and treatment duration. Long-term use of benzodiazepines should be avoided whenever possible.
(3) Patients with chronic tinnitus often exhibit specific personality traits, typically perfectionism, proneness to anxiety, and strong control needs. When faced with the inability to control their tinnitus, they can become highly anxious. Although personality traits cannot be fully altered, changing thought patterns through exercises like mindfulness meditation has been shown to modify brain function and even structure in several studies. Therefore, we recommend mindfulness practices, biofeedback, and relaxation training for these patients. This process is relatively prolonged and requires high patient adherence.

While current theories offer robust explanations for acute tinnitus, compensatory chronic tinnitus, and decompensated chronic tinnitus from both physiological and psychological perspectives, as well as elucidating various risk factors including the relationship between hearing loss and tinnitus, the transition to clinical practice presents numerous challenges. Among these are the multitude of physiological factors associated with tinnitus, many of which have high prevalence rates, making it difficult to identify and prioritize the most influential etiological factors and consequently complicating treatment strategies. Furthermore, the application of psychological interventions also confronts substantial difficulties; determining how to tailor an ideal cognitive behavioral therapy (CBT) for individual patients, and the judicious use of antianxiety and antidepressant medications, poses significant challenges that necessitate ongoing empirical experience in the clinical setting.

Before accumulating practical experience, a fundamental prerequisite is the acquisition of a sound understanding of tinnitus. This entails grounding one's approach in theoretical knowledge and proceeding to implement this in practice, sharing both setbacks and successes with patients. The iterative process of refining our comprehension of tinnitus through continuous cycles of theory refinement and practical application—where each informs and advances the other—constitutes the appropriate path forward in managing tinnitus. In essence, a synergistic, spiral progression between theoretical understanding and clinical practice is integral to advancing effective tinnitus treatment modalities.

References

1. Hoare DJ, Adjmian P, Sereda M, et al. Recent technological advances in sound-based approaches to tinnitus treatment: a review of efficacy considered against putative physiological mechanism. Noise Health. 2013;15:107–16.
2. Sweetow RW. The use of fractal tones in tinnitus patient management. Noise Health. 2013;15:96–100.
3. Engneer N, Riley J, Seale, et al. Reversing pathological neural activity using targeted plasticity. Nature. 2011;189:207–14.
4. Hallett M. Transcranial magnetic stimulation and the human brain. Nature. 2000;406(6792):147–50.
5. Biesinger E, Heiden C, Greimel V, et al. Strategien in der ambulanten Behandlung des Tinnitus [Strategies in ambulatory treatment of tinnitus]. HNO. 1998;46(2):157–69.

13 Central Sensitization Syndrome

Jilei Zhang, Qi Liu, and Lisheng Yu

In 2012, the Bárány Society proposed a definitive definition and diagnostic criteria for vestibular migraine (VM) [1], which is the most common episodic vertigo disorder [2]. VM has garnered significant attention in the field, leading to the publication of two editions of expert consensus on vestibular migraine. According to the criteria, individuals with a history of migraine who experience recurrent moderate to severe vestibular symptoms with or without headache, or those without a history of migraine but who experience 50% or more moderate to severe vestibular symptoms with accompanying migraine-like symptoms (not necessarily headache), are classified as possible VM cases. In fact, even benign paroxysmal vertigo (BPV), a condition characterized by episodic vertigo without a background of migraine, has been included as an equivalent disorder of migraine in the ICHD-3. The classification of VM as a subtype of migraine or an independent disorder remains controversial. Additionally, there is ongoing debate regarding the mechanisms underlying benign recurrent vertigo in patients who do not meet the diagnostic criteria for VM. A better understanding of the mechanisms of migraine is crucial for comprehending vestibular migraine. The pathogenesis of migraine has been a subject of prolonged debate. Initially, migraine was considered a neuronal storm, but subsequently, the theory of vascular dilation gained prominence. There are also viewpoints suggesting that migraine is a form of aseptic inflammation. With a deeper understanding of brain dysfunction, migraine is now regarded as a primary, reversible brain dysfunction disorder characterized by central sensitization. This concept is closely related to central sensitization syndrome, and migraine is one of the major diseases within the central sensitization syndrome family. This article provides a brief introduction to the concept of central sensitization syndrome and other related disorders, aiming to deepen and expand our understanding of migraine, and thereby gains further insights into common symptoms such as unexplained dizziness, ear congestion, itching, and cough [3].

J. Zhang · Q. Liu · L. Yu (✉)
Department of Otorhinolaryngology, Head and Neck Surgery, People's Hospital, Peking University, Beijing, China
e-mail: 1710301140@pku.edu.cn

13.1 History of Central Sensitization Syndrome

In 1981, Yunus first proposed the concept that fibromyalgia syndrome (FMS) [4], irritable bowel syndrome (IBS), tension-type headache (TTH), and migraine are closely related and share muscle spasms as a common feature. In 1984, Yunus described the clinical overlap between FMS, IBS, TTH, and primary dysmenorrhea and clearly depicted their interrelationships in a Venn

L. Yu (ed.), *Progress in Postauricular Administration*, Experts' Perspectives on Medical Advances,
https://doi.org/10.1007/978-981-95-5102-6_13

diagram [5, 6]. However, this viewpoint has been controversial, with a prominent question being how skeletal muscles and visceral smooth muscles are connected. In 1989, Clifford Woolf and colleagues discovered the hyperexcitability of spinal cord neurons induced by peripheral tissue injury in rat experiments, introducing the concept of central sensitization (CS). In 1993, Woolf and Chong first applied this concept clinically. In the early studies, Bennett summarized the evidence of central sensitization in FMS. In 2000, Yunus proposed that the pathophysiological mechanisms of various diseases may be related to central sensitization and classified these diseases as a family, introducing the concept of central sensitivity syndromes (CSS) for the first time. In 2007, Yunus further expanded the concept of CSS, which encompasses a series of diseases primarily characterized by central sensitization, including fibromyalgia syndrome (FMS), irritable bowel syndrome (IBS) [7], temporomandibular joint disorder (TMD), migraine, and myofascial pain syndrome (MPS), among others.

13.2 Pathophysiology of Central Sensitization

Not all members of CSS exhibit the same sensitivity to all stimuli, which may suggest heterogeneity among CSS members and indicate that central sensitization may not be the sole pathophysiological mechanism of CSS diseases. Other factors that may be related or unrelated to CSS include genetics, sympathetic nervous system overactivity, endocrine dysfunction (such as relative adrenal insufficiency and decreased growth hormone), viral infections, persistent peripheral nociceptive stimulation (such as arthritis), poor sleep, environmental stimuli (weather, noise, chemicals, adverse childhood experiences), and psychological stress. CSS is influenced by multiple factors and exhibits a multiplicative effect, wherein the combined action and interaction of several factors can amplify and sustain central sensitization and/or give rise to various syndromes. Therefore, the pathophysiology of CSS primarily involves the genetic basis, peripheral persistent pain stimulation, and the combined effects of trauma and viral infection, which result in the release of cytokines by the immune system, thereby enhancing the activity of the ascending (activating) pathways and reducing the activity of the descending (inhibitory) pathways. The resulting excessive hypersensitive response manifests clinically as pain (allodynia) in response to normal nonpainful stimuli, such as touch, and heightened pain sensitivity (hyperalgesia) in response to normal painful stimuli. Impaired descending inhibition also implies the loss of the normal process of pain inhibition, leading to secondary cutaneous allodynia (hypersensitivity of adjacent skin) and widespread hyperalgesia (hypersensitivity of distant pain). It is currently unclear whether peripheral "excessive stimulation" is necessary for the maintenance of CS. Although joint replacement surgery for osteoarthritis eliminates the pain associated with the affected joint and seems to reverse the CS process, more evidence suggests that CS is a dysfunction of spinal cord neural networks and central overprocessing, independent of persistent peripheral stimulation.

13.3 Diseases Associated with Central Sensitization Mechanism

13.3.1 Functional Gastrointestinal Disorders

The gut microbiota is a complex community that helps maintain a dynamic ecological balance. It is estimated that adults have approximately 100 trillion bacteria in their bodies, with the microbiota in the gastrointestinal tract accounting for more than 78.162% of the total microbiota. The composition of gut microbiota is not fixed and changes with age, while being influenced by various stress factors. There are significant differences in the baseline and dynamic changes of gut microbiota between individuals, and the development of gut microbiota also varies greatly between different genders. The gut microbiota and the brain are connected bidirectionally through complex neural networks, endocrine networks, and neurotransmitter networks. The neural network pathways include the enteric nervous system, also known as the "gut-brain," which is widely distributed throughout the digestive tract, the vagus nerve that connects the gut microbiota and the brain, and the central nervous system. The main function of the nervous system is to integrate incoming information, regulate gastrointestinal function, and perceive visceral sensations. This bidirectional neural communication between the brain and the gut is the applied basis of neuroanatomy and neurophysiology [7].

Various functional and organic gastrointestinal disorders, including functional dyspepsia (FD), irritable bowel syndrome (IBS), gastroesophageal reflux disease (GERD), inflammatory bowel disease (IBD), and abdominal disorders, involve mucosal stimulation and/or chronic inflammation. They involve frequent transmission of noxious neural impulses from the gastrointestinal tract to the central nervous system. The repetitive stimulation and frequent discharge of incoming nerves result in peripheral sensitization. The frequent transmission of pain signals to the central nervous system ultimately leads to central sensitization and subsequent visceral hypersensitivity, which is the mechanism underlying functional gastrointestinal disorders. Patients with IBS and those with dyspepsia often report somatic hypersensitivity and visceral hypersensitivity, which are the results of central sensitization.

13.3.2 Ear Fullness

In some cases, patients experiencing ear fullness (aural fullness) may not have excessive stimulation of the external, middle, or inner ear. Instead, their nerves or central cortical pathways may overreact to stimuli that would not normally evoke abnormal sensations, leading to the feelings of ear fullness. This phenomenon is analogous to allodynia—where nonpainful or mild stimuli trigger pain. What factors might cause hypersensitivity in neural signaling pathways [8, 9]?

In 1987, Yuasa R et al. conducted a study of 118 patients (143 ears) presenting with ear fullness as their primary complaint. All enrolled patients showed no or only mild sensorineural hearing loss, and those with middle ear disorders, vertigo, Meniere's disease, or severe cardiovascular/cerebrovascular diseases were excluded. The study revealed similarities between these patients and early-stage Meniere's disease patients in terms of age of onset, ear discomfort, and neck/shoulder stiffness. This led to the hypothesis that patients with aural fullness who had normal middle ear function and pure-tone thresholds might represent a different stage of the same disease continuum as Meniere's patients, with both conditions closely linked to autonomic dysfunction. Notably, autonomic nerve block therapy significantly alleviated ear fullness symptoms in these patients. In recent years, as understanding of vestibular migraine has deepened, many patients previously diagnosed with early-stage Meniere's disease are now recognized as likely having vestibular migraine. This suggests that idiopathic ear fullness and migraine may share common pathogenic mechanisms. In 2017, Omid Moshtaghi et al. studied 11 patients with persistent idiopathic ear fullness (average duration: 4 years) after excluding all other potential causes. These patients adhered to migraine-specific lifestyle/dietary modifications and received verapamil and amitriptyline therapy. After an average treatment duration of 5 weeks (range: 2–6 weeks), eight patients (73%) experienced significant symptom relief, strongly supporting the hypothesis of overlapping mechanisms between idiopathic ear fullness and migraine. However, only six patients (54%) in Moshtaghi's study met formal migraine diagnostic criteria [10]. This highlights the need to broaden our understanding of migraine—some patients may exhibit other manifestations of central sensitization without fulfilling classical migraine criteria.

13.3.3 Refractory Pruritus

Recent studies have shown that itch signals in the spinal cord primarily excite spinal dorsal horn neurons through ascending pathways, including nociceptive-specific neurons, wide dynamic range (WDR) neurons, and mechanically insensitive neurons, which secrete neuropeptides or neurotransmitters to transmit itch sensation. In addition, the excitatory amino acid neurotransmitter glutamate, which transmits pain signals, is also involved in the central sensitization mechanism of itch sensation. Therefore, for some chronic pruritus, especially neuropathic pruritus, drugs targeting the voltage-gated calcium channel $\alpha 2\delta$ subunit, such as gabapentin and pregabalin, can be used to reduce depolarization caused by calcium influx in nerve endings, decrease neural excitability, and regulate presynaptic neurotransmitter release, such as glutamate, to modulate neural activity. This significantly controls chronic pruritus, especially neuropathic pruritus symptoms. Additionally, itch transmission can also be regulated through descending pathways, which is consistent with the effective clinical use of 5-hydroxytryptamine norepinephrine reuptake inhibitors and other antidepressant drugs that target and modulate the descending pathways in the treatment of chronic pruritus. In some patients, there is a particularly noticeable sensation of pruritus in the ear, which may be closely related to this mechanism.

13.3.4 Vasomotor Rhinitis and Allergic Rhinitis

Vasomotor rhinitis refers to nonspecific allergic nasal hyperreactivity. There is a common neural pathway between vasomotor rhinitis and migraines, both of which are related to abnormal pain modulation pathways. There have been many studies on the relationship between allergic rhinitis and migraines. Different studies have shown that the incidence of migraines is increased in patients with allergic rhinitis, and the incidence of allergic rhinitis is increased in patients with migraines, indicating a close association between the two. In fact, early studies have shown that migraines completely resolve in patients when dietary restrictions are applied and potential allergens are eliminated, leading to the belief that "migraines are actually immune diseases." Allergic rhinitis is an IgE-mediated disease that is activated and released by mast cells and eosinophils, often leading to sinus headache. Histamine is a key mediator in the pathogenesis of allergic rhinitis and also plays an important role in migraines accompanied by nitric oxide (NO). Research has shown a close relationship between fibromyalgia (FM) and allergic rhinitis, as well as other nonallergic rhinitis. As mentioned in the previous section on central sensitization mechanism, immune abnormalities and the release of various inflammatory factors play important roles in the development of central sensitivity syndromes (CSS), and there is a mutual influence between abnormal pain processing and immune abnormalities [11–14].

13.3.5 Recurrent Sudden Sensorineural Hearing Loss

The relationship between migraines and cochlear symptoms, such as phonophobia (possibly auditory hypersensitivity), has been found to be very close. Phonophobia has been included in the diagnostic criteria for migraines. Although there is a substantial body of literature on the relationship between tinnitus, hearing loss, particularly sudden sensorineural hearing loss (SSNHL), and migraines, the exact association between them has remained unclear. In 2018, the concept of cochlear migraine was proposed, providing a clear interpretation of the relationship between recurrent SSNHL and migraines [15]. Several recent large-scale studies have demonstrated a significant association between SSNHL and migraines, with the likelihood of SSNHL occurring in the migraine group being 1.22–1.8 times higher compared to the control group [16–18]. Early studies suggested that the mechanism of migraines caused vasoconstriction in the inner ear, leading to the manifestation of SSNHL. Currently, it is believed that although vascular mechanisms are involved in the pathogenesis of migraines, migraines are primarily a brain disorder involving the trigeminovascular system, and the trigeminal nerve, through its branches, innervates the labyrinthine artery in the inner ear. Abnormally activated axons of the trigeminal nerve release neurotransmitters such as calcitonin gene-related peptide and substance P, leading to vasodilation in the inner ear. This vasodilation triggers a series of aseptic inflammatory responses, including plasma protein extravasation and tissue edema, which affect the function of the inner ear and result in the symptoms of sudden hearing loss [19–21]. This sudden hearing loss is a functional change in the inner ear under the mechanism of migraines. Therefore, the prognosis for this type of sudden hearing loss is generally good.

Our understanding of migraines should also be expanded to include other manifestations of central sensitization, even if they do not fully meet the diagnostic criteria for migraines. Thus, the concept of central sensitization is of great clinical significance in the diagnosis. Questionnaires on central sensitization have been developed abroad, covering various aspects such as chronic pain in multiple body parts, anxiety, depression, sleep disturbances, hypersensitivity to external stimuli, restless leg syndrome, chronic fatigue syndrome, temporomandibular joint disorder, irritable bowel syndrome, and others. This suggests that migraines, as a brain disorder, and the manifestations of central sensitization mechanisms behind them may involve multiple systems throughout the body. Different individuals may exhibit completely different symptoms at different times, including headache, dizziness, hearing loss, tinnitus, diarrhea, etc., which are personalized symptoms of the condition [22, 23]. Therefore, a multidisciplinary approach is needed in the diagnosis of this condition to gain a more comprehensive understanding of the manifestations of the same pathological mechanism in different systems from different perspectives. In clinical practice, when faced with patients who experience recurrent dizziness, sudden hearing loss, ear fullness, ear itching, and other symptoms, even if they do not meet the current diagnostic criteria for migraines, it is important to broaden our perspective and comprehensively evaluate whether the patients meet the criteria for central sensitization. This approach may provide a more holistic approach to diagnosing and treating the disease. Based on the literature and combined with central sensitization syndrome and the common diseases seen in our department, we have designed the following questionnaire (see Table 13.1). If two or more items are positive or if two or more items under the same category are positive, even if the patient does not meet the diagnostic criteria for migraines, it is worth considering the possibility of central sensitization and trying migraine prophylaxis treatment.

Table 13.1 Summary of symptoms associated with central sensitization syndrome

Classification	Clinical manifestations
Classification A: Hypersensitivity	Hypersensitivity to visual stimuli Hypersensitivity to visual stimuli Hypersensitivity to sound and light Hypersensitivity to odors Hypersensitivity to weather changes Hypersensitivity to medications[a]
Classification B: Family history	Family history of migraine Family history of Meniere's disease Family history of motion sickness Family history of recurrent vertigo
Classification C: Pain sensitivity	Chronic body pain History of sinus headaches History of recurrent episodes of stiff neck
Classification D: Ear conditions	Recurrent episodes of sudden deafness Chronic ear stuffiness, numbness
Classification E: Gastrointestinal conditions	Irritable bowel syndrome Gastroesophageal reflux disease
Classification F: Nasal allergy symptom	Vasomotor rhinitis Allergic rhinitis

[a]Sensitivity to multiple medications at low doses with side effects

References

1. Lempert T, Olesen J, Furman J, et al. Vestibular migraine: diagnostic criteria. J Vestib Res. 2012;22:167–72. https://doi.org/10.3233/VES-2012-0453.
2. Dieterich M, Obermann M, Celebisoy N. Vestibular migraine: the most frequent entity of episodic vertigo. J Neurol. 2016;263(Suppl 1):S82–9. https://doi.org/10.1007/s00415-015-7905-2. Epub 2016 Apr 15.
3. Colombo B, Teggi R. Vestibular migraine and related syndromes. Springer. p. 1–18. https://doi.org/10.1007/978-3-319-07022-3.
4. Yunus MB, Masi AT, Calabro JJ, Miller KA, Feigenbaum SL. Primary fibromyalgia (fibrositis): clinical study of 50 patients with matched normal controls. Semin Arthritis Rheum. 1981;11:151–71.
5. Yunus MB. Fibromyalgia and overlapping disorders: the unifying concept of central sensitivity syndromes. Semin Arthritis Rheum. 2007;36(6):339–56.
6. Yunus MB. Central sensitivity syndromes: a new paradigm and group nosology for fibromyalgia and overlapping conditions, and the related issue of disease versus illness. Semin Arthritis Rheum. 2008;37(6):339–52. PMID 18191990.
7. Jašarević E, Morrison KE. Sex differences in the gut microbiome-brain axis across the lifespan [J]. Philos Trans R Soc Lond Ser B Biol Sci. 2016;371(1688):2015–27.
8. Park MS, Lee HY, Kang HM, et al. Clinical manifestations of aural fullness [J]. Yonsei Med J. 2012;53(5):985–91.
9. Zhou E, Xiao X, et al. Studies on causes and mechanisms of ear fullness [J]. Chin J Otol. 2016;14(6):828–32. (Chinese).
10. Omid Moshtaghi, Yaser Ghavami, Hossein Mahboubi, et al. Migraine-related aural fullness: a potential clinical entity. Otolaryngology–Head Neck Surg. 2018;158(1).
11. Pattanaik D, Lieberman P. Vasomotor rhinitis. Curr Allergy Asthma Rep. 2010;10(2):84–91. https://doi.org/10.1007/s11882-010-0089-z. PMID: 20425499.
12. Güvenç IA, Acar M, Muluk NB, Kucukcan NE, Cingi C. Is there an associationbetween migraine and allergic rhinitis? Ear Nose Throat J. 2017;96(6):E18–23. https://doi.org/10.1177/014556131709600604. PMID: 28636737.
13. Ozturk A, Degirmenci Y, Tokmak B, Tokmak A. Frequency of migraine in patients with allergic rhinitis. Pak J Med Sci. 2013;29(2):528–31. https://doi.org/10.12669/pjms.292.3148. PMID: 24353570; PMCID: PMC3809225.
14. Frieri M, Argyriou A. Is there a relationship between fibromyalgia and rhinitis? Allergy Asthma Proc. 2012;33(6):443–9. https://doi.org/10.2500/aap.2012.33.3596. PMID: 23394501.
15. Lai JT, Liu TC. Proposal for a new diagnosis for cochlear migraine. JAMA Otolaryngol Head Neck Surg. 2018;144(3):185–6. https://doi.org/10.1001/jamaoto.2017.2427.
16. Chia-Huei Chu, Chia-jen Liu, Jong-ling Fuh. Migraine is a risk factor for sudden sensorineural hearing loss: a nationwide population-based study. Cephalalgia. 2013;33(2):80–6. https://doi.org/10.1177/0333102412468671. Epub 2012 Nov 28.
17. Hwang JH, Tsai SJ, Liu TC, et al. Association of tinnitus and other cochlear disorders with a history of migraines. JAMA Otolaryngol Head Neck Surg. 2018;144(8):712–7. https://doi.org/10.1001/jamaoto.2018.0939.
18. Kim SY, Kim MK, Lim JS, Kong IG, Choi HG. Migraine increases the proportion of sudden sensorineural hearing loss: a longitudinal follow-up study. Auris Nasus Larynx. 2019;46(3):353–9. https://doi.org/10.1016/j.anl.2018.10.006. Epub 2018 Oct 30.
19. Virre ES, Baloh RW. Migraine as a cause of sudden hearing loss. Headache. 1996;36:24–8. https://doi.org/10.1046/j.1526-4610.1996.3601024.x.
20. Lee H, Lopez I, Ishiyama A, Baloh RW. Can migraine damage the inner ear? Arch Neurol. 2000;57:1631–4. https://doi.org/10.1001/archneur.57.11.1631.
21. Arslan Y, Arslan İB, Aydin H, Yağiz Ö, Tokuçoğlu F, Çukurova İ. The etiological relationship between migraine and sudden hearing loss. Otol Neurotol. 2017;38(10):1411–4. https://doi.org/10.1097/MAO.0000000000001617.
22. Mayer TG, Neblett R, Cohen H, Howard KJ, Choi YH, Williams MJ, Perez Y, Gatchel RJ. The development and psychometric validation of the central sensitization inventory. Pain Pract. 2012;12(4):276–85. https://doi.org/10.1111/j.1533-2500.2011.00493.x.
23. Luzeiro I, Luís L, Gonçalves F, et al. Vestibular migraine: clinical challenges and opportunities for multidisciplinary [J]. Behav Neurol. 2016.

Insights on Benign Paroxysmal Positional Vertigo (BPPV)

14

Nishan Chen and Lisheng Yu

The repositioning treatment for BPPV is simple, easy, and effective, representing a milestone in the treatment of vestibular diseases and promoting the rapid development of vestibular medicine. As knowledge of this disease spreads, clinicians from various departments related to dizziness have shown great enthusiasm and recognition for this condition. Our hospital started dealing with this disease in 2006, and over 10 years, we have manually repositioned thousands of cases. Here are a few insights to share:

14.1 What If the Repositioning Treatment for BPPV Is Ineffective After Repeated Attempts?

In outpatient clinics, I often encounter patients whose repositioning at other hospitals was ineffective. It is undeniable that for some patients, the repositioning technique was improper, leading to poor results. However, this accounts for only a small proportion, especially for patients who have undergone repositioning three times or more by experienced doctors; this situation is even rarer. More often, the nystagmus characteristics in patients are not prominent, raising the question: Does nystagmus during positional testing always indicate BPPV? When I first encountered this disease in 2006, I was most concerned with the repositioning technique and was surprised by its effectiveness. Around 2010, as the number of patients increased, many patients exhibited nystagmus during positional testing that did not align with the characteristics of BPPV. Many showed very mild, persistent nystagmus, leading to the proposal of the concept of atypical BPPV. I also wrote articles on this subject, debating why nystagmus should sometimes be typical and sometimes atypical if it is caused by canaliths floating in the semicircular canal or adhering to the cupula. At that time, a concept was also proposed: benign paroxysmal positional vertigo (BPPV) is a symptom diagnosis, whereas otolithiasis is its mechanism, and there may be different mechanisms behind the same symptoms, which could be the source of atypical BPPV. This discrepancy might be due to translation issues, as discussed in the chapter on "Some Views on Professional Translation's Fidelity, Conveyance, and Elegance." Since this terminology is now conventionally accepted, distinguishing BPPV with noncanalith mechanisms from those with canalith mechanisms is essential. The 2017 Guidelines for Diagnosis and Treatment of Benign Paroxysmal Positional Vertigo (BPPV) by the *Chinese Journal of Otorhinolaryngology Head and Neck Surgery* proposed the concept of diagnostic grading, including definitive diagno-

N. Chen · L. Yu (✉)
Department of Otorhinolaryngology, Head and Neck Surgery, People's Hospital, Peking University, Beijing, China

L. Yu (ed.), *Progress in Postauricular Administration*, Experts' Perspectives on Medical Advances,
https://doi.org/10.1007/978-981-95-5102-6_14

sis, possible diagnosis, and controversial syndromes. By understanding the diagnostic grading concept, it becomes clear that some patients with positive positional tests but poor repositioning outcomes might not be experiencing BPPV due to canalith mechanisms, apart from a few cases with technique issues.

14.2 What Proportion of Controversial Syndromes Is There? What Are the Characteristics of the Nystagmus?

For this question, we conducted clinical observations and published our findings in both Chinese and English clinical otorhinolaryngology journals [1, 2].

The incidence rate of controversial syndromes in BPPV: the first statistical analysis included 113 patients with positive positional nystagmus, totaling 121 instances. The proportion of nystagmus conforming to definite BPPV accounted for 40.5% (49/121). The second analysis included 243 patients with positive positional nystagmus, excluding those with sudden hearing loss, Ménière's disease, and vestibular neuritis, with 65% (159/243) conforming to definite BPPV nystagmus. Hence, diagnosing BPPV solely based on nystagmus during positional tests could lead to a misdiagnosis rate of up to 50%. If BPPV is diagnosed solely based on patient complaints of dizziness upon movement, the misdiagnosis rate is even higher.

Compared to the definitive diagnosis group, the controversial group showed no abnormalities in saccade tests, smooth pursuit, or optokinetic nystagmus tests. The duration of nystagmus in the controversial group was generally over 1 min, often accompanied by spontaneous nystagmus and post-head-shaking nystagmus. The horizontal nystagmus intensity in the controversial group was weaker than that in the definitive diagnosis group for horizontal canalith BPPV, while the vertical nystagmus intensity was weaker than that in the posterior canal BPPV, with statistically significant differences. To summarize, the nystagmus characteristics in the controversial group primarily included spontaneous nystagmus, post-head-shaking nystagmus, nystagmus duration >1 min, and weaker nystagmus intensity.

Chi-square tests showed no significant differences between the two groups regarding histories of recurrent dizziness, headaches, or motion sickness. The main differences in medical history between the two groups were twofold: first, the prevalence of headaches is significantly higher in the controversial group, with statistically significant differences. Second, the proportion of silent brain infarction is notable. Among the 121 instances, 69 cases (57%) were referred to the otolaryngology department from related departments (such as the emergency department, neurology, and orthopedics), after undergoing head CT or MRI examinations. Among these, 22 instances found small silent infarction lesions, diagnosed by specialists as previous conditions unrelated to the current onset. Of these 22 patients with silent brain infarction, 19 belonged to the controversial syndrome group, and only 3 belonged to the definitive diagnosis group.

14.3 What Are the Pathological Mechanisms of Controversial Syndromes in BPPV?

The results of these two studies indicate that the controversial group may be related to the following three possible mechanisms.

14.3.1 Light cupula

In the second study, among the 243 patients with positive positional nystagmus, 15 had a light cupula. The concept of a light cupula was initially proposed in the context of alcohol-induced positional nystagmus, primarily because alcohol diffusion into the cupula and endolymph alters their density and specific gravity. The nystagmus of a light cupula has the following characteristics:

(1) When the head is turned approximately 25° to the affected side in the supine position, a null point can be observed.

(2) Nystagmus toward the affected side appears when the head is tilted forward 90°, and horizontal nystagmus toward the healthy side appears during the head-back or supine test.
(3) The roll test and head-tilt test can induce direction-changing positional nystagmus (DCPN), which lasts more than 1 min without latency and fatigue.

Currently, the mechanism for light cupula is unclear. It may be due to a reduced density of the cupula or increased density of the endolymph, resulting in a density difference between the two. The reasons for reduced cupula density may be related to the intake of glycerol and alcohol, cupula atrophy or swelling, or adherence of lighter substances, possibly due to some underlying diseases and allergic reactions causing changes in cupula characteristics. Another factor receiving attention is the impact of migraines on the inner ear. The sensory innervation of the middle ear and inner ear is different, with the middle ear innervated by the mandibular nerve from the trigeminal ganglion and the inner ear by the ophthalmic branch of the trigeminal nerve. Theoretically, inflammation from recurrent migraine attacks can affect the characteristics of the cupula, causing cupula atrophy and reduced density. Therefore, the migraine mechanism cannot be ignored in the occurrence of a light cupula. Increased endolymph density is related to the increased secretion of large molecules and inflammatory proteins. Kim et al. found mild bleeding and increased protein density in the inner ear of sudden deafness patients. Due to the disruption of the blood-labyrinth barrier, plasma proteins and other substances from the inner ear vessels infiltrate the endolymph, increasing its specific gravity. Thus, sudden deafness is also one of the mechanisms causing a light cupula.

14.3.2 Migraine-related positional vertigo

The mechanism of central positional nystagmus is currently unclear but is hypothesized to be related to lesions in the dorsolateral fourth ventricle, the dorsal part of the cerebellar vermis, and the cerebellar nodulus and uvula. In normal physiological states, the midline structures of the cerebellum primarily integrate signals from the otolith organs and semicircular canals, controlling the otolith-ocular reflex and participating in semicircular-ocular reflex regulation. When the midline structures of the cerebellum are dysfunctional, the integration of signals from the otolith organs and semicircular canals is impaired, leading to abnormal central velocity storage, which induces central positional nystagmus. Migraine is the most common disease causing central functional abnormalities. Literature reports that 19% of vestibular migraine patients have spontaneous nystagmus, and 35% have post-head-shaking nystagmus. Vestibular migraine positional nystagmus is characterized by low speed and duration that does not conform to nystagmus induced by a single semicircular canal. Vestibular migraine is one of the most common vestibular disorders, with a prevalence of 1.5–5 times higher in women than in men, affecting 1% of the general population or 11% of patients visiting dizziness clinics. In this study, the composition ratios of women in the definitive diagnosis group and the controversial syndrome group were 79.6% and 77.8%, respectively, significantly higher than that of men in both groups. The nystagmus intensity varied significantly between the two groups, with the controversial group mainly exhibiting low-frequency, low-speed nystagmus.

14.3.3 In this study

There was a significant difference in the number of patients with brain infarction lesions between the two groups based on head CT or MRI results. Among the 69 patients referred from other departments who underwent cranial imaging, 22 had small lacunar brain infarcts, with 19 in the controversial syndrome group and only 3 in the definitive diagnosis group. Although these lacunar infarcts could not be confirmed as the responsible brain infarcts for dizziness and nystagmus, they suggest that patients in the controversial syndrome group may have underlying central lesions. These underlying lesions may not be severe but could affect the complex network functions of the central nervous system. First, white matter damage generally involves the subcortical tracts, leading to cortical-subcortical disconnection syndrome, causing gait instability and loss of balance. Additionally, the frontal and prefrontal lobes have rich neural projections to the vestibular nuclei, known as the "vestibular cortex." Damage to the white matter in the frontal and prefrontal lobes can impair vestibular functions, leading to sensory and motor dysfunctions and dizziness. Although no research has yet confirmed the relationship between minor brain infarcts and positional nystagmus, further research on central functions may provide answers.

The results of this study show that the proportion of controversial syndromes is indeed not low. Diagnosing all positional nystagmus as BPPV would generalize the diagnosis of BPPV. In diagnosis, it is crucial to remember the characteristics of BPPV nystagmus, and only those matching the characteristics can be diagnosed as BPPV. Otherwise, other potential mechanisms should be thoroughly considered. The light cupula and migraine mechanisms are currently more widely accepted, but there is still much exploration space for other mechanisms.

14.4 What Are the Precautions for Repositioning in Confirmed BPPV Cases?

For the confirmed diagnosis group, the repositioning technique does not present significant technical difficulties. The main challenges are first to confirm whether BPPV is indeed caused by a canalith mechanism and how to handle abnormal situations during repositioning.

Regarding the first point, it is very important to remember the nystagmus characteristics confirming the diagnosis of BPPV: the direction of nystagmus should be consistent with the plane of the semicircular canal; there should be a certain latency period; it should last for a certain time; it should show fatigue; opposite movements should produce nystagmus in the opposite direction; and the nystagmus should show a gradual increase and then decrease, with particular attention to the last two points. If the positional nystagmus does not conform to these characteristics, repositioning can be attempted, but it should be understood that it is likely not a canalith mechanism, and the repositioning might not be effective. There is no need for repeated attempts. However, even if the nystagmus characteristics perfectly match, the repositioning process may not always be smooth.

14.4.1 For posterior canal BPPV

If a second same-direction nystagmus appears during the Epley maneuver, it generally suggests effective repositioning, especially important for patients with strong nystagmus. When handling such patients, if no second same-direction nystagmus appears during the first repositioning, I increase the height of the pillow, making the head tilt more pronounced, and extend the waiting time for each movement during the second repositioning. This prevents different canalith clusters from moving at different speeds, thereby increasing the success rate. If unsuccessful, I perform the head-shaking test to change the starting position of the canalith and reattempt the repositioning after resting for half an hour to an hour. If other types of nystagmus are induced after repositioning, what should be done? If the nystagmus can be localized to a canalith displacement, it is often due to canal switching during repositioning, and repositioning can continue. However, if the nystagmus is difficult to explain and localize, the best approach is to "stop." Ask the patient to perform home exercises and provide symptomatic medication, and then review in 3 days. During the review, the patient's nystagmus might either disappear or become more typical, allowing for targeted repositioning. Since this is a benign condition, inducing repeated vertigo without a specific treatment method is detrimental. Observation and recovery are also good treatment methods. The prerequisite of the "stop" approach is that it must already be confirmed as a benign condition.

14.4.2 For horizontal semicircular canal BPPV

During testing, try to make the patient turn over rather than just turning the head, as sometimes the head-turning angle is insufficient. Determining the affected side is challenging. I prefer to observe nystagmus while the patient is lying flat, turning over toward the nystagmus direction and judging the canalith type and side based on the nystagmus after turning over. I also use intensity-based judgment. Clinically, a situation frequently occurs where the patient shows no nystagmus when turning to one side but shows nystagmus when turning to the other side. Which side is the affected side in this situation? It might not necessarily be the side with nystagmus. As mentioned before, for a confirmed diagnosis of BPPV, opposite movements should produce opposite-direction nystagmus. When this situation does not appear, it cannot be judged. Based on my experience, after repeated inductions, the side without initial nystagmus is often the affected side. In my view, unexplained nystagmus is more common in horizontal semicircular canal repositioning than in posterior canal BPPV. Frequently, the initial supine position shows nystagmus in one direction, but after repositioning, the nystagmus direction changes, making intensity and direction hard to explain. My approach remains twofold: either perform the head-shaking test and reexamine after a rest or conduct recovery exercises and review after 3 days.

14.4.3 For horizontal canal light cupula BPPV

Although it is commonly seen clinically, converting from a light cupula to a canalith using the Gufoni maneuver is not frequent. Some instructors believe it might be due to insufficient head-shaking force. Careful observation reveals that converting to a canalith does not require much force. In some elderly patients concerned about cervical spine issues, I do not perform the Gufoni maneuver but simply have the patient turn over quickly several times in bed, resulting in switching from ageotropic to geotropic nystagmus. This suggests that in some patients with horizontal canal light cupula BPPV, other mechanisms may be at play.

14.4.4 For anterior canal BPPV

Firstly, it is quite rare. Over the years, I have confirmed less than ten cases. One patient left a deep impression: repeated repositioning three times was ineffective until the fourth time, when posterior canal BPPV nystagmus appeared, making the repositioning very effective. Therefore, I believe in the existence of pseudoanterior canal BPPV (i.e., canalith settling at the shared crus of the anterior and posterior canals). The reason why canalith sits in that location remains unexplained.

14.5 How to Treat Controversial Syndromes in BPPV? Is Repositioning Still Required?

Based on our team's experience, the answer is yes. Repositioning treatment is simple: clinical experience suggests that whether the positional dizziness is migraine-related or some light cupula patients, even if nystagmus changes are not apparent, the subjective feeling of dizziness can sometimes be reduced. Brain function is very complex, and repeated inductions of dizziness might promote the central nervous system's adaptation to dizziness or restart the central balance system. Considering the benefits to patients and their effort, attempting repositioning is definitely worthwhile. However, if 1–2 attempts do not yield results, there is no need for repeated attempts.

Even without trying repositioning again, continuing recovery exercises is still recommended to promote the central adaptation to positional vertigo. Patients can continue home Brandt-Daroff recovery therapy, usually requiring 50–60 repetitions a day, which can be done in multiple sessions or in one go.

14.6 Should Controversial Syndromes Be Treated with Medication? What Medication Is Appropriate?

For confirmed BPPV, medication is not recommended unless symptoms are particularly severe, making repositioning intolerable or if residual dizziness appears after repositioning, requiring some medication. For the controversial syndromes group, corresponding medication treatment is needed. The basis for medication treatment is the pathogenesis. If the understanding of the disease changes, the treatment will naturally change. Controversial syndromes might be related to migraines, allergic reactions, or sudden hearing loss; the treatment direction is naturally toward these mechanisms. Nevertheless, research in this area is scarce. Based on literature and our team's experience, the migraine mechanism is an important cause of controversial syndromes, thus requiring antimigraine treatment. Since most patients' nystagmus is not strong and dizziness is not severe, flunarizine and betahistine are recommended. Sibelium is a guideline-recommended migraine preventive medication, while betahistine can reduce vestibular nerve excitability, providing symptomatic relief to some extent. For severe symptoms, diphenidol is recommended. Both light cupula and migraine-related positional vertigo have a self-healing tendency, so symptomatic treatment combined with rehabilitation gradually alleviates patients' symptoms. Although the average nystagmus intensity in our study's controversial syndrome group was only 7°/s, indeed low-frequency low-speed nystagmus, some patients, especially those with light cupula, may experience stronger nystagmus intensity and more severe symptoms. For these patients, Fei Li conducted an observational study in "Clinical Characteristics of Positional Vertigo with Ineffective Repositioning and Negative MRI" documenting that initial nystagmus types were divided into horizontal ageotropic (53.49%, 23/43), horizontal geotropic (6.98%, 3/43), vertical downbeat (9.30%, 4/43), and mixed (30.23%, 13/43). Randomized grouping showed that 21 patients (48.84%) received clonazepam treatment, while 22 patients (51.63%) received flunarizine hydrochloride treatment. The average maximum slow phase velocity (SPV) before treatment was 56°/s for the enrolled patients, with no difference between the groups. After 3 days of medication, the maximum SPV of the clonazepam group significantly decreased compared to the flunarizine hydrochloride group, indicating a significant difference. Thus, clonazepam treatment for acute positional nystagmus with ineffective repositioning and negative MRI was more effective than flunarizine hydrochloride. Clonazepam might have a therapeutic effect on central positional nystagmus by enhancing the cerebellar inhibitory signal output. For patients with frequent attacks (more than twice a month or lasting more than 3 days per episode in 2 months) and ineffective repositioning for positional dizziness, preventive treatment with Sibelium for 2 months significantly reduced the average number of dizziness attacks per month compared to the control group. I have used this method clinically for patients with strong nystagmus and controversial BPPV syndromes but should be cautious of clonazepam's side effects, especially in older adults.

To date, there is no clinical guideline or targeted clinical trial for cerebral small vessel disease (CSVD). Thus, there is no specific medical treatment method for CSVD. For asymptomatic CSVD, lifestyle adjustment is recommended rather than medication. Since dizziness is a transient disease and small vessel disease is a slowly progressive condition, the two are not directly causal but are high-risk factors. For these patients, rehabilitation treatment should be strengthened, including both balance recovery and cognitive rehabilitation.

14.7 How to Manage Refractory BPPV?

First, what is considered refractory BPPV? How many times should repositioning be performed? How long should treatment be ineffective before being considered refractory? For controversial group patients, positional nystagmus caused by light cupula and migraine may need 2–4 weeks to disappear; such patients might have a longer treatment cycle but are not refractory. If the confirmed group undergoes more than three repositionings and nystagmus persists, it is indeed rare but possible. For some patients, nystagmus changes in every examination suggest it might not be a confirmed group case. In any case, rehabilitation is the best treatment method. Performing Brandt-Daroff rehabilitation can not only facilitate the dissipation of possible canaliths but also promote central habituation. Similar to medication, rehabilitation exercises must reach a certain dosage to be effective. For refractory cases, I usually require 50–60 repetitions a day, which can be done in multiple sessions or in one go. For general BPPV, I usually recommend about 30 repetitions, with 6–8 repetitions per session.

14.8 How to Understand the Mechanism of Residual Dizziness After Repositioning? How to Manage It?

Several studies show that 48–72 h after successful repositioning treatment, unsteadiness and feeling "light-headed" occur with an incidence rate of 36.6–61%, defined as residual dizziness (RD). It manifests as nonpositional, nonrotational, persistent lightheadedness and unsteadiness, with the most common symptom being lightheadedness (63%) and floating sensation as the second most common. We also conducted a statistical study on this topic, dividing RD into mild RD and severe RD based on its impact on daily life, with occurrence rates of 21 of 44 (47.7%) and 10 of 44 (22.7%), respectively, totaling 70.4% [3]. Scholars have conducted many studies on RD mechanisms, mainly focusing on physiological mechanisms: first, a small amount of otoconia that cannot cause vertigo but might cause lightheadedness; second, otoconia returning to the utricle, altering its input, requiring the central nervous system time to adapt to the change; and lastly, extensive peripheral vestibular system lesions, which still cause imbalance even after successful repositioning. However, analyzing these possible mechanisms carefully, if otoconia fragments float in the endolymph, even in small amounts, the produced dizziness should be positional. The currently accepted RD standard is nonrotational, nonpositional lingering dizziness. The second mechanism suggests adaptation related to otoconia returning to the utricle; however, adaptation in otolith organ pathology typically takes only 3 days. Natural history studies on RD show most patients' residual symptoms disappear in 20 days.

It is suspected that the physiological mechanism might not be the primary reason; other mechanisms such as psychological factors might be more significant. Psychological factors greatly influence dizziness. There is a mutual influence between vestibular diseases and psychological disorders; the proportion of psychological disorders in dizziness patients is 5–15 times higher than in the general population, and psychological pressure gradually increases in patients with a long history of BPPV, requiring sufficient attention. Psychological construction during repositioning is important, explaining to patients the possibility of RD during repositioning, so they do not become overly anxious and exacerbate the feeling of dizziness when RD symptoms appear.

Additionally, two patients who experienced RD were advised to perform home rehabilitation exercises. One patient reported dizziness becoming significantly worse when moving from lying to sitting but not from sitting to lying. They were referred to cardiology and ultimately diagnosed with orthostatic hypotension. Literature shows that among successfully repositioned BPPV patients, at least 35% had abnormal tilt table tests and orthostatic hypotension, with those in the RD group having a significantly higher rate. Comparing RD and non-RD groups, orthostatic hypotension incidences were 43% and 3%, respectively. The vestibulospinal reflex aids in maintaining blood pressure stability during postural changes.

Finally, comprehensive examination is still required; some patients might have concurrent central tumors, necessitating careful exclusion.

Understanding the mechanism of residual dizziness allows targeted management and treatment.

14.9 What Are the Factors for BPPV Recurrence?

In 2020, a graduate student from our department conducted a meta-analysis on this topic [4], resulting in 4076 search results, with meta-analysis including 60 articles producing 24 results. The risk factors for BPPV recurrence include female gender, age (65 years old), hyperlipidemia, diabetes mellitus, hypertension, migraine, cervical spondylosis, osteoporosis, head trauma, otitis media, abnormal vestibular-evoked myogenic potentials, and prolonged computer use. No significant differences were observed concerning the involved semicircular canal's side, type, smoking, alcohol intake, stroke, ear surgery, dizziness duration before treatment, repositioning attempts, Ménière's disease, sleep disorders, hypercholesterolemia, and 25-hydroxyvitamin D levels. These results suggest that BPPV is multifactorial, making it difficult to identify a clear cause, posing challenges in prevention. However, if it is typical BPPV, the recurrence probability is generally more than half a year, with effective repositioning, making aggressive preventive treatment unnecessary. If patients experience frequent episodes, based on migraine history, ginkgo biloba extract or Sibelium may be given for 1–2 months; however, no statistical analysis exists for the preventive effect, and such patients are rare in my clinic.

Understanding any disease is easy to start but difficult to master. Although we have significantly expanded and deepened our understanding of BPPV in recent years, many questions remain worth further exploration.

References

1. Yunjuan L, Xiaoqin WU, Haijun S, Xin MA, Lisheng YU, & Rencong L, et al. Analysis of nystagmus and medical history of 121 patients positive with positional test. Journal of Clinical Otorhinolaryngology Head and Neck Surgery. 2018.
2. Lin Y, Xue J, Su-Jeong Lee, Wu X, & Jen-Tsung Lai. Value of clinical data and positional testing in patients with positional vertigo. Clinical otolaryngology: official journal of ENT-UK; official journal of Netherlands Society for Oto-Rhino-Laryngology & Cervico-Facial Surgery, 2019;44(6).
3. Wang Yuguang, Zhang Yanqing, Liu Yan, et al. Changes in the Dizziness Handicap Inventory before and after successful repositioning in patients with idiopathic benign paroxysmal positional vertigo. Chinese Journal of Otology, 2018;16(3):6. DOI: CNKI:SUN:ZHER.0.2018-03-008.
4. Shichang, Li, Zijing, Wang, Yan, Liu et al. Risk Factors for the Recurrence of Benign Paroxysmal Positional Vertigo: A Systematic Review and Meta-Analysis.[J] .Ear Nose Throat J, 2020, 101: NP112-NP134.

MIX
Papier aus verantwortungsvollen Quellen
Paper from responsible sources
FSC® C105338

If you have any concerns about our products,
you can contact us on
ProductSafety@springernature.com

In case Publisher is established outside the EU,
the EU authorized representative is:
Springer Nature Customer Service Center GmbH
Europaplatz 3, 69115 Heidelberg, Germany

Printed by Libri Plureos GmbH
in Hamburg, Germany